Well-being in the Early Years

CRITICAL APPROACHES TO THE EARLY YEARS

You might also like the following books from Critical Publishing

Teaching Systematic Synthetic Phonics and Early English
Jonathan Glazzard and Jane Stokoe
978-1-909330-09-2 In print

Teaching and Learning Early Years Mathematics: Subject and Pedagogic Knowledge
Mary Briggs
978-1-909330-37-5 September 2013

Early Years Policy and Practice: A Critical Alliance
Pat Tomlinson
978-1-909330-61-0 September 2013

The Critical Years: Early Years Development from Conception to 5
Tim Gully
978-1-909330-73-3 January 2014

Most of our titles are also available in a range of electronic formats. To order please go to our website www.criticalpublishing.com or contact our distributor, NBN International, 10 Thornbury Road, Plymouth PL6 7PP, telephone 01752 202301 or e-mail orders@ nbninternational.com.

Well-being in the Early Years

Caroline Bligh, Sue Chambers,
Chelle Davison, Ian Lloyd, Jackie Musgrave,
June O'Sullivan and Susan Waltham

CRITICAL
APPROACHES
TO THE EARLY
YEARS

First published in 2013 by Critical Publishing Ltd

The authors have made every effort to ensure the accuracy of information
contained in this publication, but assume no responsibility for any errors,
inaccuracies, inconsistencies and omissions. Likewise every effort has been
made to contact copyright holders. If any copyright material has been reproduced
unwittingly and without permission the Publisher will gladly receive information
enabling them to rectify any error or omission in subsequent editions.

Copyright © 2013 Caroline Bligh, Sue Chambers, Chelle Davison, Ian Lloyd, Jackie
Musgrave, June O'Sullivan and Susan Waltham

British Library Cataloguing in Publication Data
A CIP record for this book is available from the British Library

ISBN: 978-1-909330-65-8

This book is also available in the following ebook formats:

Kindle ISBN: 978-1-909330-66-5
EPUB ISBN: 978-1-909330-67-2
Adobe ebook ISBN: 978-1-909330-68-9

The rights of Caroline Bligh, Sue Chambers, Chelle Davison, Ian Lloyd, Jackie
Musgrave, June O'Sullivan and Susan Waltham to be identified as the Authors of
this work have been asserted by them in accordance with the Copyright, Design
and Patents Act 1988.

Cover and text design by Greensplash Ltd
Project management by Out of House Publishing
Printed and bound in Great Britain by TJ International Ltd

Critical Publishing
152 Chester Road
Northwich
CW8 4AL
www.criticalpublishing.com

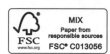

MIX
Paper from
responsible sources
FSC® C013056

Contents

Meet the authors

Caroline Bligh leads and teaches across several master's and undergraduate Initial Teacher Education modules in the School of Education and Childhood at Leeds Metropolitan University. She is a qualified teacher and State Registered Nurse, with a particular research interest in English as an Additional Language.

Sue Chambers has spent her professional life working in the early years sector, first as a nursery nurse; then as a teacher, working in nursery schools and classes in areas with high levels of social deprivation; and then as head of a nursery school. Since then she has worked as an early learning adviser for a local authority, and as a freelance consultant.

Chelle Davison is a Senior Lecturer of Early Years Professional Practice at Leeds Metropolitan University. Her role incorporates developing the critical understanding of early years pedagogy and its practical application in settings and schools. Chelle has recently made significant contributions to a range of policy documents and government reviews, and is a devoted supporter of the professionalisation of the early years workforce.

Ian Lloyd is a Lecturer in Social Work at Staffordshire University.

Jackie Musgrave is a Senior Lecturer at the University of Worcester. She qualified as a sick-children's nurse and then taught in a college of further education for 16 years. She has a master's degree in early childhood education from the University of Sheffield and is currently studying for her doctorate. Her research looks specifically at how practitioners create inclusive environments for children from birth to age three with chronic conditions.

June O'Sullivan, MBE is Chief Executive Officer of the London Early Years Foundation (LEYF), one of the UK's largest childcare charity social enterprises. With 350 staff across 24 community, workplace and Children's Centre nurseries in six key London boroughs, LEYF is dedicated to building a better future for London's children, families and local communities.

Susan Waltham is a Senior Lecturer teaching on a number of undergraduate and postgraduate courses in the School of Education and Childhood at Leeds Metropolitan University. Her academic expertise is in child psychology and human development, diversity and equality. Her research is centred on identity construction in young children in multicultural, multilinguistic settings.

Acknowledgements

'Does day care damage your baby?' Lucy Cavendish. Reproduced on pp 43 and 44 © Telegraph Media Group Limited, 2011.

Introduction to critical thinking

What is critical thinking?

This introduction gives you the opportunity to learn more about critical thinking and the skills you will acquire as you use this series, introducing you to the meaning of critical thinking and how you can develop the necessary skills to read and research effectively towards a critical approach to learning and analysis. It is a necessary and wholly beneficial position to be starting with questions and finishing your journey with more questions.

> *Judge a man by his questions rather than by his answers.*
> François-Marie Arouet (Voltaire)

If you are already a professional within the early years sector, maybe as a teacher in a Reception class, or as an early years educator in a private day-care setting, you will no doubt have faced many challenging debates, discussions at training events and your own personal questioning of the policies faced by the sector as a whole. We want you to ask these questions. More importantly, we believe it to be an essential and crucial part of your professional development. You will no doubt be required to implement policies that might at first seem detached from your day-to-day professional practice. It is critical that you question these policies, that you understand their purpose, and moreover that you understand how they have come into being.

Often students are faced with complex definitions of critical thinking that require them to deconstruct the concept before they fully understand just how to 'do' the critical thinking in the first place. For example,

> *Critical thinking is the intellectually disciplined process of actively and skilfully conceptualizing, applying, analysing, synthesizing, and/or evaluating information gathered from, or generated by, observation, experience, reflection, reasoning, or communication, as a guide to belief and action.*
> (Scriven and Paul, 1989)

Rather than confusing you with specific academic definitions, it is our hope that as you read further and begin to understand this topic more, you will be encouraged to ask contemplative questions. Alison King emphasises the importance of students acquiring and cultivating a *habit of inquiry* to enable them to *learn to ask thoughtful questions* (King, 1995, p 13). Contrary to the standard methods of 'instruction' that leave the student as a passive recipient of information, King argues that where a student has developed the skills of critical thinking they become an 'autonomous' learner:

> *Such a habit of inquiry learned and practiced in class can be applied also to their everyday lives: to what they see on television, read in the newspaper observe in popular culture and hear during interaction with friends and colleagues, as well as to decisions they make about personal relationships, consumer purchases, political choices, and business transactions.*
>
> (King, 1995, p 13)

Consider the subject matter that you are now researching; you may have been tasked with the question 'How has policy changed over the past 25 years?' This is what King would suggest is a 'factual' question, one that may well have a limited answer. Once you have this answer, there is a tendency to stop there, making the inquiry fact-based rather than critical. If you were to follow up this first question with a critical question, King would argue that you are beginning to 'introduce high level cognitive processes such as analysis of ideas, comparison and contrast, inference, prediction [and] evaluation' (1995, p 140)

Example

Factual question	Critical question
How has policy changed over the past 25 years?	What has been the impact of policy change over the past 25 years?
Which policies have been introduced to support childcare and early education initiatives recently?	How has childcare and early education been influenced by recent policy?

Critical thinking has been described by Diane Halpern (1996) as

> *thinking that is purposeful, reasoned, and goal directed – the kind of thinking involved in solving problems, formulating inferences, calculating likelihoods, and making decisions when the thinker is using skills that are thoughtful and effective.*
>
> (Halpern, 1996)

The emphasis is on 'thinking' that alludes to the student pausing and considering not only the topic or subject in hand, but also the questions generated from taking an opportunity to ask those critical rather than factual questions.

To think critically signifies the ability to use 'a higher order skill' that enables professionals to act in a rational and reasonable manner, using empathy and understanding of others in a specific context, such as an early years setting. The rights and needs of others are always the priority, rather than blindly following established procedures.

A critical thinker:

* raises vital questions and problems, formulating them clearly and precisely; gathers and assesses relevant information, using abstract ideas to interpret it effectively;

* reaches well-reasoned conclusions and solutions, testing them against relevant criteria and standards;

* thinks open-mindedly within alternative systems of thought, recognising and assessing, as need be, their assumptions, implications and practical consequences;

* communicates effectively with others in figuring out solutions to complex problems.

(Taken from Paul and Elder, 2008)

Alec Fisher (2001) examines the description given by John Dewey of what he termed *reflective thinking* as *active, persistent and careful consideration of a belief or supposed form of knowledge in the light of the grounds which support it and further conclusions to which it tends*. Rather than rushing to discover what you believe to be 'the answer', consider disentangling the question and the 'right answer' before stating your conclusion. Could there be more to find by turning your factual question into a critical question?

Below are examples of a student discussing her recent visit to another early years setting. The first question is what King (1995) describes as a factual question, and you can see we have highlighted exactly where the facts are in the answer. The second question is a critical question (King, 1995), and again we have highlighted in the answer where the critical elements are.

Question (factual):

What did you see in the new setting that is different to your setting?

> *The equipment that was out didn't seem a lot [FCT], in my setting we have everything out [FCT] so the children can access it all, you know like continuous provision. In the other setting they had bare shelves [FCT] and they told me that new equipment was only brought out when the children had mastered those already out [FCT]. They didn't seem to be bothered about the EYFS either, like nothing in the planning was linked to the EYFS [FCT].*
>
> (Early childhood studies student, 2013).

Question (critical):

Consider the two different approaches, your setting and the one that you visited. What impact do you think they have on the children's learning and developing?

> *I suppose I can see that when we put toys and materials out, that there are always children who get things out but don't have a clue how to use it. I guess it would be better if there was less and that the things they did get out were right for the developmental level of each child [CRIT]. I suppose it is how we interpret continuous*

provision [CRIT]. I think as well that the other setting was using the EYFS to measure the development and learning of each child [CRIT], but they knew the framework and the children well enough not to have to write it all down all the time [CRIT].

(Early childhood studies student, 2013).

Another example of how you can become a critical thinker might be in asking yourself critical questions as you read and research a topic.

Thought provoking or critical questions require students to go beyond the facts to think about them in ways that are different from what is presented explicitly in class or in the text.

(King, 1995, p 14)

Stella Cottrell (2005) suggests that we must know what we think about a subject and then be able to justify why we think in a certain way *having reasons for what we believe ... critically evaluating our own beliefs ... [and be] able to present to others the reasons for our beliefs and actions* (Cottrell, 2005, p 3).

Five questions towards critical thinking

1. Do I understand what I am reading?

2. Can I explain what I have read (factually)? For example, what is this author telling me about this subject?

3. What do I think? For example, what is my standpoint, what do I believe is right?

4. Why do I think that way (critically)? For example, I think that way because I have seen this concept work in practice.

5. Can I justify to another person my way of thinking?

All that we ask is that you take the time to stop, and consider what you are reading:

What a sad comment on modern educational systems that most learners neither value nor practise active, critical reflection. They are too busy studying to stop and think.

(Hammond and Collins, 1991, p 163)

We encourage you to take time to ask yourself, your peers and your tutors inquisitive and exploratory questions about the themes discussed in this book, and to stop for a while to move on from the surface-level factual questioning for which you will, no doubt, only find factual answers, and to ponder the wider concepts, the implications for professional practice, and to ask the searching questions to which you may not find such a concrete answer.

For as Van Gelder so eloquently suggests, learning about it is not as useful as doing it:

For students to improve, they must engage in critical thinking itself. It is not enough to learn about critical thinking. These strategies are about as effective as working on your tennis game by watching Wimbledon. Unless the students are actively doing the thinking themselves, they will never improve.

(Van Gelder, 2005, p 43)

Introduction: challenging assumptions and misconceptions about well-being in the early years

It is generally accepted that a child's well-being is determined by numerous factors. In much the same way that an adult's well-being is affected by external influences such as working arrangements, financial security, domestic relationships and educational attainment (Strazdins et al., 2011; Conti and Heckman. 2012; Li et al., 2012). It is often assumed that professionals are striving to work together, interprofessionally and within a multi-agency framework. The assumption, evidenced by the chapters in this book, is correct to a certain extent.

> *Everyone who works with children – including teachers, GPs, nurses, midwives, health visitors, early years professionals, youth workers, police, Accident and Emergency staff, paediatricians, voluntary and community workers and social workers – has a responsibility for keeping them safe.*
>
> *No single professional can have a full picture of a child's needs and circumstances and, if children and families are to receive the right help at the right time, everyone who comes into contact with them has a role to play in identifying concerns, sharing information and taking prompt action.*
>
> *In order that organisations and practitioners collaborate effectively, it is vital that every individual working with children and families is aware of the role that they have to play and the role of other professionals.*
>
> (DfE, 2013b, p 8)

The chapters in this book highlight just how various professionals view a child's well-being. An early years teacher steps back from her daily coaching of a small student in her class, allowing the child to become more autonomous in her learning (Chapter 1). A health professional sees importance in ensuring that the environment a child resides in throughout their school or nursery day is appropriate and inclusive of their complex medical needs (Chapter 2). A parent leaves their child in the hands of a professional that they trust, irrespective of whether that is a teacher, a doctor or a social worker; parents want to know their child is eating and sleeping well, that they have had fun (Chapter 3).

Each professional with responsibility for a child has their own views on what constitutes support for a child's well-being. Without question, professionals are entirely focused on the well-being of children; however, they are focused on that task from within their own profession.

There is a significant difficulty in moving from one's own profession across to another, something that is essential in order for interprofessional working to be successful.

> *Multi-agency working is about different services, agencies and teams of profession-als and other staff working together to provide services that fully meet the needs of children, young people and their parents or carers. To work successfully on a multi-agency basis you need to be clear about your own role and aware of the roles of other professionals; you need to be confident about your own standards and targets and respectful of those that apply to other services, actively seeking and respecting the knowledge and input others can make to delivering best outcomes for children*
>
> (DFES, 2004, p 18, in Trodd and Chivers, 2011)

The collection of perspectives in this book shows clearly that each professional is relatively secure in their expertise, yet they are caught in a world dominated by their own subject and vocational area of expertise. This, we believe, is representative of the various sectors as they do their very best to put children at the centre of their professionalism and desire for a better future for every child and family. Irrespective of the subject area, every professional has, without question, been predisposed to centre their care, learning, professional development and personal experiences on the children they protect and serve.

In trying to ensure that the very best is done for each child, a professional might not view the child's world as a bigger canvas that requires many colours to create a perfect picture. In the throes of dealing with a child protection issue, does the social worker see the perspective of the early years teacher? In the chaos of an Ofsted inspection does an early years educator consider the perspective of a health professional? All too many serious case reviews cite a lack of professional continuity between the various sectors surrounding each child: educational professionals not working cohesively with health professionals, whose paperwork then fails to find the social worker.

We are not writing this book to lay criticism at the feet of any of the professions; neither can we criticise the amazing and detailed work of each professional represented here. Nonetheless, the model created by Community Care (see Figure 1) is all too often the reality of multiprofessional working. Each individual professional eagerly doing their job, playing their part and leaving the child in the centre feeling a little disillusioned, detached and, like their parents, a little confused as to who is doing what.

This text asks you as the reader to consider each perspective, and to try to understand, unpick and critically evaluate just how we all work together in the best interests of each child whom we are privileged to represent. It is no coincidence that every serious case review cites problems in communicating the needs and experiences of our youngest children; we would simply like you to consider just how difficult it really is to ensure that everyone who needs to know about a child actually knows about that child.

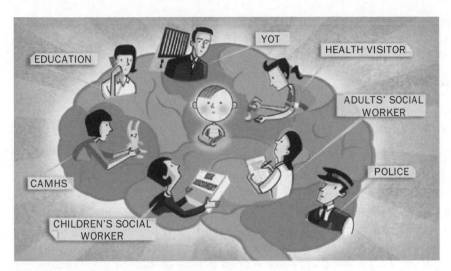

Figure 1 Community Care, 2011

The passion we have as professionals in our own field of expertise allows us little time to explore how other professionals feel and think about their own area. How often have we sat and explored a scenario with a professional from a different field? When was the last time you asked a doctor, a nurse, a health visitor, a teacher, an early years educator or a parent what they think of a specific situation or example of practice? I imagine the answer, as for us, is either 'I haven't' or 'not for a very long time'.

We are so passionate about the roles we play in the pursuit of a better life for all our children, we do forget to stop, to chat, to discuss and debate, then to go home and reflect on that time. So, as you navigate this book you will read about the passion and eagerness of all the various professionals who place children at the centre of their daily work. You will hear stories, read examples and come to understand the theoretical background that has become the bedrock of children's professionals.

Do not assume as you read these chapters that you will complete your own studies or further your own career and miraculously have the time to ensure you have acknowledged, studied and involved each professional who needs to have important information at their disposal in order to support a family or help a child successfully.

Do not assume that you will 'make time' to learn more about the other sectors that are different from your own, that you will be guaranteed to come across colleagues from these other areas of the early years professions, or that you will even stop to consider 'who else do I need to speak with?'.

This is not to say that we as professionals have not improved over time to allow for a multiprofessional approach to serious concerns of child protection or family matters. Since the death of Victoria Climbié in 2000 and Baby P in 2007, there have been huge improvements made across the country in multiprofessional working. Indeed, you may well find yourself involved in a variety of meetings where the intense needs of a child are at the centre of discussions: where decisions might well be made based upon your own observations of children and their family.

We draw your attention not only to your own role within the care, education and protection of children, but also to the reality that to be part of a truly multiprofessional team is far more difficult than it seems.

Critical question

» How easy is it for each area of care and education to come together?

CASE STUDY

Emily's story

I went to a parents' evening to see my little girl's Year 1 teacher. Despite her being at the top of her class, despite her working in the Year 2 classrooms for maths and other subjects because she was able, her Year 1 teacher said nothing positive. We knew that she did well. Don't get me wrong, we don't have a child genius on our hands, but she is an able child who can be stretched a little. We thought that following her Reception year and a report that contained the comment 'model student' from the head teacher that we would be hearing how hard she had worked to stay at the top of her class. We thought we would be told she had a positive attitude to school and that she had been a pleasure to teach. We were devastated by the comments of her teacher:

'She can't sit still, she can't concentrate, she fidgets, she messes with her shoes and anything that is in reach, she could do better, she knows the answers to questions but I don't know how because she never listens.' This was not the report we had expected from her Year 1 teacher.

It was hard for me especially. I know enough about early brain development to know that a six-year-old cannot sit still. Their brains are busily making connections around phys-ical development and so they jig and fidget almost constantly. I know that some children go through this phase at five and others at seven. I know that those connections are reinforced around eight, and at that time they are made a permanent part of their brain development. I asked the teacher if she would consider giving her a button, a piece of Blu-tack or another small object to hold in her hands during the carpet time, when the teacher expected the children to sit still. I knew that, while her brain was busy and occu-pied by the spinning of a coin or the squeezing of the Blu-tack, she would sit still and be able to concentrate on the maths or phonics being taught via smart board.

The teacher's answer baffled me; maybe shocked would better describe it: 'But then they'd all want something to play with.' I remember pausing for a few seconds that seemed to last hours, thinking 'Of course they will all want something; they're all at a similar stage in their brain development. How does she not know this? Surely teachers of young children know how their brains are wiring and how they learn best?'

I left wondering if I should change the school my children were attending, or if I could help them to understand the processes of movement development. What could I do?

As a parent I began to realise just how detached teachers really are: professionals who hold such power and control over such tiny, young developing minds and yet have little or no knowledge of how their brains work. The gap between parents and teachers made me consider the health visitors who rarely and seemingly randomly knocked on my door: health professionals who had seen only two of my four children in the nine years I'd been a parent. I realised it was a gap that existed in many areas of child-orientated professions. I was the parent; where were the professionals designated to care as much for my child's well-being as I was? As a parent I'm on my own, and I can't be an expert in health, education, social care and parenting.

Where were the professionals to help me?

(Emily, 34)

We believe there is an assumption that being multiprofessional is something everyone is striving for. We believe that there is a misconception on the part of early years professionals in all areas of care and education that becoming multiprofessional comes with time and experience. It does not. As professionals we must stand in the shoes of a social worker who struggles to explain to an adult that they have a four-year-old half-brother, or in the shoes of a health visitor who is told by a parent that their child will not be having the new two-year-olds' developmental check. How do we know just how to communicate effectively if we have never taken time to consider the perspective of that professional?

Frameworks for well-being

We do not have to look very far to see an array of frameworks that represent the complexity of children's well-being. Whichever you decide to use in the course of your learning is likely to represent how you envisage the various elements of a child's life coming together.

Bronfenbrenner (1979) provided the theoretical model behind the development of Sure Start during the New Labour era of the 1990s and early 2000s. The model essentially considers all individuals as active agents in the development and alteration of their environment; however, he reasoned that the external environment in which an individual lives also has an intense impact upon the behaviours of that individual and of those around them. This might explain how a child's well-being is influenced through the use of external childcare, or family commitment to educational experiences, or the impact of poverty of aspirations within the home (see Figure 2). Other child well-being models – some used to assess risk – include the child model devised by Redcar and Cleveland Children and Young People's Trust (see Figure 3).

It is essential that, while you consider each perspective, you also consider the children from more affluent families, two-parent families and those who do not meet the poverty criteria. In 2010 Waldfogel et al. identified that one-fifth of children in the US were born into single-parent households and that a further fifth resided in homes where two unmarried adults cohabited (Waldfogel et al., 2010): too often the children who are born under the label of single-parent household, or to the stigmatising marker of a teenage parent, are the individuals where well-being is considered most. What about children who have the nice house on the leafy green estate in the suburb of a town or city, where they go to a small church school and have two working parents? These children may not be a target for an assessment of their overall well-being, and yet they may very well be in need of support or intervention. Would you see a child in need if they lived in an affluent area?

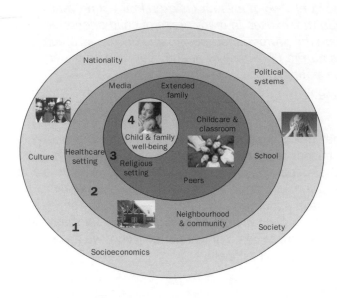

4 Microsystem: for example, the playgroup, pre-school education, childcare or childminder setting where the child actively experiences a particular pattern of events, roles and interpersonal relationships.

3 Mesosystem: interrelations between two or more setting in which the child actively participates – for example, home and nursery, childminder and playgroup.

2 Exosystem: settings that do not involve the child as an active participant but in which events occur that affect, or are affected by, what happens in the micro-systems – for example, local authority systems or inspection structures.

1 Macrosystem: historical/social/ cultural/ecological environments at national policy level.

Figure 2 Influences on a child's well-being at a number of levels. Adapted from Anning and Hall 2008 & Centre for Child and Family Wellbeing

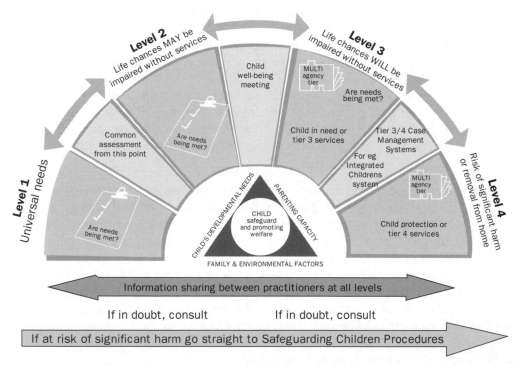

Figure 3 Child well-being model by Redcar and Cleveland Children and Young People's Trust

The professional is you

Each chapter in this book is taken from a slightly different perspective. Everyone is none-theless consumed by their desire to improve and maintain the well-being of children. Each professional does that in a slightly different way; some may visit the homes of young children, others see children from 9am until 3.15pm and others collect their children from settings needing only to put them to bed. No one is wrong in their approach, and everyone would hope that they could work effectively with the other professions in order to guarantee the very best for the child. A parent attempting to ensure they have the right work–home balance feels compelled to spend 'quality time' with their children (Milkie et al., 2010). A teacher on a weekend feels compelled to visit a child in their home environment to encourage their speech and language skills inside the classroom. The child being at school from 7.30am to 6.30pm is acceptable to the parent despite only having weekends free. The teacher is eager to help the child who is often away from home. The discontinuity and seeming incoherence between the desires of a parent and the determination of a teacher may give rise to feelings of inadequacy in the parent and exacerbate the feelings of control by the teacher. The slight-est change in that power relationship tips the balance to favour a parent or tips it to favour the teacher. Relationships between each professional and the child are tentative and evolu-tionary, ever hanging in a cyclic model of repetitive behaviours and misunderstandings.

What is more important to you? And to a parent?

A tea stain on a child's vest three school days in a row?

A child who is writing pages of beautiful descriptive writing about their trips to the woods after school with their father, who shows them a variety of animals, birds and growing plants?

A parent's and a child's teacher's understanding of a child's well-being may well be very different. A social worker's understanding of a child's well-being can be very different from that of an early years educator.

We have brought together some perspectives on children's well-being. In one book you can read for yourself and hear the determination each professional has to 'get it right'. There is not one who is more right, or one who is more important. Each perspective is valid and essential to the well-being, success and security of each individual child.

Each perspective highlights just how intensely professionals work within their own area of expertise, thus proving the difficulty in stepping outside their own daily interactions to see, and really know, the importance of another's perspective.

We challenge you to set aside any assumptions or misconceptions that you may have regard-ing the view that 'all professionals work together'. In theory that is exactly what we need to be doing, and yet parents still feel shunned by teachers, and teachers are so busy that they run out of time to consider the child who has worn the same summer dress for so long that there is now half a metre of snow on the ground.

It will be a challenge for you to keep your own personal views and preconceptions separate from your chosen career: how you have been raised and your own experiences of schooling, as well as your adult familiarities, will all come together, forming your preconceived views of the world around you. You will already have an idea of how you think things 'should be' for a child. What we are tasking you with is to consider the variety of different views and perspectives, untainted by your own bias. This would be a challenge for even the most seasoned professional; nevertheless it is worth your undertaking this stimulating process of thought and action.

The well-being of a child can be defined in numerous ways (see below); even within this text, professionals all use the term to mean something slightly different, and all use it within the context of their own field of expertise. You must decide what well-being means to you. We set you the challenge to learn more about each professional who works for and with our youngest children across the world.

Definitions of well-being

* FreeDictionary.com: well-being (wĕl'bē'ĭng) *n.* The state of being healthy, happy, or prosperous; welfare.

* Pollard and Lee (2003) refer to well-being as *a complex, multi-faceted construct that has continued to elude researchers' attempts to define and measure it.*

* Statham and Chase (2010) term well-being as *the quality of people's lives. It is a dynamic state that is enhanced when people can fulfil their personal and social goals. It is understood both in relation to objective measures, such as household income, educational resources and health status; and subjective indicators such as happiness, perceptions of quality of life and life satisfaction.*

Statham and Chase (2010, p 2) go on to state that the definition of well-being – particularly childhood well-being – is not only complex but *multi-dimensional, [and] should include dimensions of physical, emotional and social well-being; [it] should focus on the immediate lives of children but also consider their future lives; and should incorporate some subjective as well as objective measures.*

If, as professionals, we are still trying simply to define what we all mean by children's well-being, then it surely follows that across the professions, and arguably within each profession, work is carried out differently, and with more subjectivity than objectivity, on a daily basis. Our own interpretation of what we mean by well-being, and what we deem to be of importance to ensure children's well-being, is very likely to be different from that of our colleagues both inside and outside our chosen profession.

It is not denied that each of us strives to deliver the very best for the children we work with; however, can we safely say we are truly multiprofessional in our approach to ensure the well-being of our nation's children?

How are each of the perspectives on well-being relevant?

It is important that as you read each chapter, you keep in the forefront of your mind the one consistent thread of continuity that links each perspective, that:

> the well-being of the child is central to each professional and the work that they do, each perspective is grounded in the desire to meet every need a child may have and to ensure their ultimate and entire well-being.

Critical questions

As you continue to explore each chapter consider some important critical questions.

» *Are there comparisons to be made between each chapter and, if so, what are they and how can the comparisons help you to understand why a child's well-being is important to the professional involved?*

» *Each professional intends to support, improve and guarantee the well-being of each child. How they do this differs between each profession. How can the boundaries between each profession be made flexible enough to allow for a multiprofessional approach to a child's well-being?*

» *The individual chapters are symbolic and representative of the separation that occurs between each perspective on well-being. Consider your own perceptions of well-being and reflect upon your own profession; which chapter do you identify with and how might you improve the flexibility of boundaries between your own perspective and that of another?*

Critical thinking chapter by chapter

Don't forget to apply your critical thinking skills as you reflect on each chapter. As you read about Suki (Chapter 1), consider the actions of the teacher and how those actions resulted in a child who had previously been silent in class, suddenly having the confidence in her teacher, and her environment, to begin to engage verbally with her peers and with her teacher. What drove a Reception class teacher to knock on the front door of one of her pupils? How would that action be seen today in 2013? Could you envisage yourself ever considering visiting the home of a pupil?

The overall and entire well-being of one silent, Reception class pupil was of utmost importance to her teacher. As you learn more about Suki and her teacher, you may well reflect on your own experiences in classrooms or with groups of children.

I read this chapter days before attending my first sports day, not as a teacher but as a parent. As I proudly searched the lines of excited children, my eyes became fixed upon a teacher and a small, frail-looking child whose ethnic origin and culture at home resonated with me and my reflections on Suki, whose first language was not English. The teacher picked up a tiny little girl who appeared terrified of her immediate surroundings and of the football she was expected to kick. Her teacher held her tightly around her chest and swung the child's legs out in front pushing the football as she stepped across the tracks. When you consider the findings of this chapter you are likely to be forever aware of the Suki in your classroom, and the impact a teacher can have on the well-being of a child.

Each chapter provides you with an example of how different professionals deal with the well-being of a child. You have the opportunity to compare the practices of each professional at the same time as making your own judgement on the successes, and failures, of your own experiences and the professionals themselves. We encourage you to be critical of the case studies within each chapter, and to question how the professional maintains and improves the well-being of each child and their family.

It is essential that you ask critical questions throughout each chapter, and we have provided you with some questions to support your own critical evaluations. As you contemplate each case study and each chapter, you should move forward with three critical points:

1.   each chapter provides an individual perspective from a professional within the early years sector on the well-being of a child;

2.   each perspective will differ depending on the role this professional plays and we have brought this to the forefront of critical discussion as it is an imperative consideration when trying to build multiprofessional approaches to working with children;

3.   every professional agrees without question, that the overall well-being of a child is of paramount importance.

You will learn as you explore the chapters that what is important to a parent is no less important to the teacher; however, it is almost impossible for a teacher to think like a parent while they are playing the role of a teacher in a school. Equally, the aspects of well-being that are almost inarguable to a social worker, are of less consequence to the parent who thinks nothing of putting a child to bed after a day at the beach where meals have consisted of little more than sugar and fats. Ice cream, doughnuts and candy floss can be seen in very different ways when considered within the role of a parent, or the role of a social worker.

These stark contrasts and differences all contribute to the problems faced by professionals who are trying, and indeed told, to work in a multidisciplinary, multiprofessional manner, where individuals are required to step outside of their day-to-day role and consider another professional and their role in achieving positive well-being for a child.

We hope that by providing you with an individualised account of each professional and their case studies, you will be able to identify the areas where a multiprofessional approach would be beneficial. However, no less importantly we want to provide an example of just how difficult it can be to do that. As we await the publication of yet more serious case reviews, and the decision of government on the overhaul of early years services and curricula, will you be thinking about 'who to blame' or will you consider the examples given within these few chapters, showing that every professional has the interests, safety, health, education and well-being of every individual child securely at the centre of their actions, decisions and professional role?

How will you bring everyone's perspectives together?

1 An early years teacher's perspective on silent participation

CAROLINE BLIGH

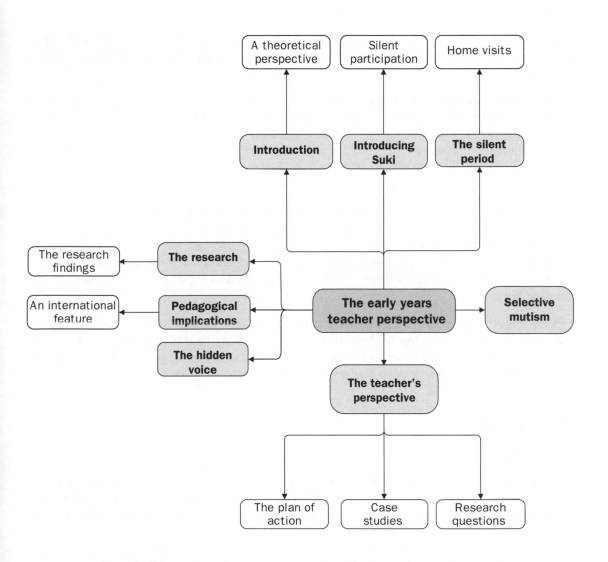

Introduction

Well-being may have been considered a subjective notion in the years prior to the Children's Society's unique research (2012a, b) that has deepened our understanding of well-being in relation to young children's learning and development.

The *Promoting Positive Well-being for Children* report states that *school is a key area of children's lives where experiences vary greatly and negative experiences have a significant impact on well-being* (Children's Society, 2012a, p 6). This key document states that *children who felt they had been unfairly treated by their teacher on more than one occasion were four times more likely to have low levels of happiness at school than children who did not feel unfairly treated.*

The *Good Childhood Report* supported these findings, revealing that *school is viewed as a central component of overall well-being by children*, and that of particular importance is *satisfaction with the school environment, relationships with teachers and other children at school, and school work and learning* (Children's Society, 2012b, p 39).

This chapter provides the reader with a case study through which to consider the well-being of a young bilingual learner in relation to her learning and development in an early years setting.

Drawing upon sociocultural research (Bligh, 2011), the reader is called upon to examine the emergent stage of English language acquisition, the *silent period*, through the silent experiences of a four-year-old girl of Japanese heritage called Suki. The silent period (in this research) refers to a specific time in the acquisition of English as an Additional Language, when, on entering an early years setting in England, the language of discourse and instruction (English) is not understood.

Suki, who has entered an English-speaking early years setting, is an emergent bilingual learner. The terms *silent, young bilingual learner*; *emergent bilingual learner*; and *English Additional Language learner* commonly refer to a young child between three and six years of age who is in the initial (non-verbal) stage of additional-language acquisition. Suki is learning English as a new and additional spoken language within and beyond the early years educational setting.

This case study aims to challenge your thinking as you are invited to 'listen in' on Suki's silent experiences. In attempting to unravel the complexity of the silent period, you will share this narrative account of Suki while she negotiates her learning trajectory through the English-speaking practices presented in the early years setting – a Reception class. I was Suki's Reception class teacher.

CASE STUDY

Introducing Suki

While teaching, I first encountered Suki as a four-year-old girl of Japanese heritage in a Reception class in a large city in the north of England. She did not speak in class, neither had she in the day nursery that she had previously attended for two years. My perception of Suki at that time was that of a 'bewildered' child, whose facial expression appeared to remain 'fixed' and unsmiling at all times. Her limbs were held stiffly and her movements appeared restricted. To my dismay the children would lift Suki's arms up and down and say *Look, Suki is just like a doll!*

Within the Reception class, spoken English was both the language of instruction (spoken by myself) and the primary spoken language of the majority of Suki's peers. Indeed, most teachers and early years practitioners in England are monolingual English speakers. Regardless of their heritage language (mother tongue), children in England are taught through the medium of spoken and written English in and through all curriculum areas in both the Early Years Foundation Stage (EYFS) (DfE, 2012b) and the Primary National Curriculum (DfE, 2012a).

Unfortunately, in the misguided belief that nurturing more than one language puts a child at a disadvantage in the development of their spoken English, the child's mother tongue may be disregarded in school, or even be actively discouraged. However, in Wales and Scotland there is less emphasis on integration into spoken English; both Welsh and Gaelic are supported in their development as indigenous languages alongside spoken English.

Silent participation at home and school

... before we left Suki's house for the ten-minute walk to school, Suki showed me her Japanese lunch box with all its beautifully sectioned compartments that contained a selection of her favourite foods. As we passed the front of Suki's house in the direction of school, she proudly pointed out the Japanese radishes that were growing in her garden, while both she and her mother attempted to converse with me (in English). Throughout the journey Suki was holding my hand. However, as soon as the school gates came into view, Suki let go of my hand and 'stiffened up'. Her face became almost 'mask-like' and she stopped speaking. Her mother and I both attempted to converse with Suki, but there was no response from her until she left the school building at 3.15pm.

At home, Suki was an adept and confident speaker in her mother tongue. However, Suki was a novice and newcomer to the (English) language awaiting her within the boundaries of the school environment. From the moment the school was in sight, Suki stopped speaking and appeared as if concentrating hard – to gain mastery of the school's unfamiliar practices and make meaning of her new world.

Unwittingly in class, I focused my attentions intensely upon Suki in an attempt to 'tease' her out of her silence and 'include' Suki as a central character within the Reception class practices. I would not only impose my gaze upon Suki and constantly ask questions of her, but also actively encourage her to participate in activities presented on the interactive white board and to present her completed pictures and models to the rest of the class. However, Suki did not want to be a central character, and preferred to seek out safe spaces that provided her with a secure 'look-out post' from which to absorb the practices of the class. As confirmed by Lave and Wenger, Suki required *lessened intensity, lessened risk, special assistance, lessened cost of error, close supervision, or lessened production pressures* (Lave and Wenger, 1991, p 100).

Suki was not withdrawing from participation when she released my hand as we walked closer towards the school gates. On the contrary, she was drawing upon her unspoken mother tongue (Vygotsky, 1978, pp 56–57) as a tool through which to observe closely and listen intensely to the practices within the early years setting. Suki watched and listened to the Reception class practices, but her participation remained limited within the confines of the school.

In contrast to school, Suki's home was surrounded with known and shared cultural signs, symbols and tools that empowered her not only to practise spoken English, but also to 'rehearse' increasing levels of participation – without feeling pressured to do so. Suki's home provided her with safe domestic spaces (Hancock and Gillen, 2007) through which to rehearse the unfamiliar practices of the early years setting – through which to learn.

During one of my visits to Suki's home, I observed her playing 'schools'. She appeared happy as I watched her at play, rehearsing the practices that she had observed and listened to in class. One such activity was Suki acting out the role of a Reception class teacher. I observed her reading a story to and asking questions of the 'children', which in reality were her dolls and soft toys. Suki's home provided her with the necessary security, cultural knowledge and agency through which to participate with confidence. Her concentration on learning the practices of the early years setting was reflected through this active role of apprenticeship (Rogoff, 1990, p 90). Actively copying what she had seen in class was of great importance to Suki as a means to increase her participation.

Akin to Lave and Wenger's description of how newcomers gradually build sketches of the practices within a learning community (1991, p 95), Suki's experiences at home and school were a means to 'sketch' participation – as a sociocultural practice.

The silent period

Not every young bilingual learner encounters a silent period like Suki, because not every child invests many of their hours, days, weeks and years in an environment where their mother tongue may be disregarded (Bligh, 2011).

A diagnosis of *selective mutism* – an extremely complex expressive communication disorder (SMIRA, 2007) – is sometimes confirmed as little as *one month* into the silent period. In fact, some Education Authority Ethnic Minority Achievement Services advise teachers that *it is crucial children are diagnosed and treated as early as possible* (HEMAS, 2003, p 2).

Although there is much conflicting information regarding the acceptable length of time within which a young bilingual learner should experience the 'silent period' or 'silent phase', many researchers (Clarke, 1996; Tabors, 1997) view the experience of passing through the silent period as a normal stage in additional-language acquisition. It is suggested by Tabors (1997) that silence is chosen because the bilingual learner prefers to communicate non-verbally. Saville-Troike's study into private speech described this period as *linguistic development that has gone underground* or, if the child is using private speech (speaking only to themselves), *social speech that has turned inward* (Saville-Troike, 1988, pp 568, 570).

Many factors may or may not have an effect upon the speed at which a child passes through the silent period, including the consequences of psychological withdrawal or an interruption in the child's expected *language acquisition processes* (Parke and Drury, 2001). Kagan (1989) suggests that children who are temperamentally inhibited will be more cautious, less sociable and perhaps less willing to try; they may be fearful (with no one to share their mother tongue) of making a mistake, therefore prolonging the transition through the silent period.

At that time I was initially concerned with the complexity of Suki's experiences that might be restricting her participation in the Reception class collaborative learning activities. Of particular concern was whether this prolonged period of silence might position her as an 'outsider' (Lave and Wenger, 1991) and restrict her from sharing 'insider' participation. For this reason I referred her to the speech and language therapist in an attempt to articulate her 'condition'.

The speech and language therapist interpreted Suki's silence as selective mutism. She referred Suki to the educational psychologist. After 'interviewing' Suki (she remained silent throughout) for approximately 20 minutes, the educational psychologist gave a confirmed diagnosis of this anxiety-based disorder.

At that time, I was relieved that a medical diagnosis had been achieved for Suki, because I assumed that a diagnosis would help solve her 'problem'. Suki's mother was also happy that a reason for Suki's silence had been established. However, I soon came to realise that pathologising Suki with a condition disregarded not only sociocultural factors affecting her whole person (Engel, 1980) but also labelled her negatively … as a deficit medical model (McConkey and Bhurgri, 2003).

Reflecting upon this episode in Suki's life-world, I realise I had unwittingly treated her with benign neglect, because I was accepting the medicalisation of Suki's silence. A deficit medical model (labelling) provided a quick-fix solution (programme of treatment) and, more importantly, a just reason for accepting Suki's behaviour as a condition. Following on swiftly from her initial diagnosis as a 'selective mute', a stimulus-fading programme of treatment (Croghan and Craven, 1982) was prescribed by the educational psychologist. Something that has disturbed me greatly is how quickly, on diagnosis, a child like Suki can be relabelled solely on the basis of their condition. Rather than being a girl with specified barriers to her learning and participation, Suki was now the *selective mute*.

At this time, the relevance of *my position* in Suki's learning was beginning to emerge. How could I, a white, monolingual (English-speaking) teacher, bridge-build between Suki's familiar 'world of home' and the unknown and possibly distrusted 'world of the school'? But, how, as a white, monolingual, adult English speaker, was I to interpret silent experiences when I was unable to share the signs, symbols and tools embodied within the young learner's mother tongue? How could I make the intangible tangible?

Home visits

After gaining consent from the head teacher of the school and Suki's mother it was agreed by all parties that I should begin visiting Suki in her home twice a week before school to try and re-establish 'new beginnings' between the school, Suki and her family.

When I visited Suki in her home, she 'came alive'.

At 8.30am, when I first arrived at Suki's house, I was met at the door by a very different girl from the four-and-a-half-year-old girl (of Japanese heritage) that I had encountered in my Reception class. Suki appeared at the door as animated and smiling. She immediately greeted me by jumping up and down, saying excitedly, 'Mrs Bligh, Mrs Bligh!' She held my hand and guided me quickly through the hall. Suki's mother welcomed me in, opened the door to the lounge and offered me a seat ... I found it hard to believe that Suki (who was now singing happily in her mother tongue) was the same young girl who would remain 'motionless' and silent in my Reception class. She brought me her school reading book, sat next to me, and attempted to read it to me in English.

Among the family's culturally shared signs, symbols and tools, Suki chatted to me with excitement and showed me her favourite toys. She walked happily with me to school, holding both my hand and that of her mother until she was in sight of the school gates: at which point her speech and facial expressions froze – and did not 'thaw' again until she left the school gates at the end of the day.

I can only imagine the initial frustration felt by Suki at being unable to draw upon and present her wealth of social, historical and cultural understanding – her *funds of knowledge* (Moll et al., 2005) – through which to make meaning of her new world. Moll et al. (1992, p 133) interpret funds of knowledge as *the historically accumulated and culturally developed bodies of knowledge and skills essential for household or individual functioning and well-being*. Teachers/practitioners may be guilty of neglecting bilingual learners' rich cultural and cognitive resources nurtured within home environments, and therefore overlook valuable opportunities for culturally responsive and meaningful teaching and learning practices.

Selective mutism

I return to Suki's 'diagnosis' in attempting to differentiate between selective mutism and the silent period. What is this condition that was attached to Suki?

Afasic UK defines selective mutism as referring to children who are able to speak freely in some situations but do not speak in others. The 'problem' presents in school where there are concerns that a child has not spoken for two terms or more (Afasic, 2004, Glossary 6).

The school speech and language therapist who had observed Suki had described selective mutism as an expressive language or communication disorder, while the educational psychologist referred to selective mutism as a psychiatric, anxiety-based condition. Speech Disorder UK (2010) suggests that selective mutism occurs when a child who has the ability to both speak and understand language fails to use this ability in some settings – the child appears to freeze and be unable to speak.

Afasic UK (2004) provides an introductory 'picture' of selective mutism.

• Selective mutism is a relatively rare condition; the best estimate suggests that fewer than 1 child per 1,000 is affected.

• Selective mutism is usually reported between the ages of three and five years.

• Girls are affected slightly more frequently than boys.

- Children who come from a bilingual background are slightly more likely to display selective mutism.

- Children with selective mutism are more likely to have other speech and language difficulties than other children.

- The majority of children with selective mutism are of average or above-average intelligence, but some show moderate-to-severe learning difficulties.

What is of particular significance to this inquiry is that not only are bilingual learners considered more likely to display selective mutism (Cline and Baldwin, 2004), but the age at which it is usually reported (between the ages of three and five years) corresponds with that at which children usually attend an early years setting.

Siraj-Blatchford and Clarke (2003) articulate the silent period as a time when some young children who are learning a new and additional language in a strange environment do not talk, describing the features these children present as:

- refusal to interact in any way or be included in interactions;

- initially no use of non-verbal behaviours;

- reluctance to respond with gestures or eye contact;

- rejection of interaction with other children or staff;

- reluctance to speak (may also be in first language);

- difficulties in settling into the nursery or school.

(Siraj-Blatchford and Clarke, 2003, p 49)

The above features described as normal for a young child passing through the silent period are remarkably similar to those characterising selective mutism. Cline and Baldwin (2004) ascribe the higher incidence of selective mutism in bilingual learners to sociocultural dissonance resulting from the incongruity of belonging to two cultures, and the need to learn a new and unfamiliar language. Perhaps Drury (2007) is nearer the 'truth' when suggesting that silence is a chosen agentive strategy. Sage and Sluckin (2004) add that a child may feel isolated if there are no children or adults in the class who speak their mother tongue. Perhaps feelings of isolation cause the spoken word to start turning inwards?

The teacher's perspective

Through the 'lens' of the educational psychologist, Suki appeared to be presenting with a set of 'symptoms' that required 'fixing'. What concerned me at that time (and still does) is why *Suki* was perceived as the 'problem'.

To 'facilitate' Suki's learning I:

- constantly focused my attention upon Suki;

- encouraged (unsuccessfully) her full participation;

- sat her by my side during whole-class delivery of information;

- sat next to her when she had a writing task;

- walked her up to the interactive white board;
- held her attention through eye contact when calling the register;
- asked the children to clap Suki whenever she engaged in an activity.

Critical questions

Suki's prolonged period of silence raises three critical questions in relation to the medicalization of children in early years settings. Examine the following.

» *Draw upon theoretical sources from social psychology to analyse critically the discrepancies between Suki's silent experiences and those of an early years teacher.*

» *Applying a sociocultural theoretical framework, evaluate the consequences of presenting a deficit medical model in relation to Suki's meaning-making during the silent period.*

» *Re-evaluate the key pedagogical implications for early years teachers in relation to government policy and current early years practice.*

The plan of action

However, following from my regular visits to Suki's house (participating in her life-world) I began to make meaning of the institutional constraints impinging on Suki's ability to negotiate her way through the silent period. I therefore decided to 'back off' from 'forcing her hand' into participation.

Instead I:

- lessened my focus of attention on Suki;
- allowed her to sit at the back of the carpet (no longer in front of me);
- no longer sat next to her when she was 'on task';
- no longer brought her up to the interactive white board;
- moved on when calling the register without expecting a response from her;
- allowed her to mediate her fractionally increasing participation;
- discouraged children from clapping Suki if she 'performed'.

In assisting Suki to gain confidence and attempt participation I decided to make some other changes too. Firstly I gave Suki's mother a tape recorder to use at home so that Suki could be recorded reading her schemed reading book. Her mother would return it to class each day and I would play it back so as to hear Suki read. I could then change her reading book accordingly, which allowed Suki to progress with her reading alongside her peers.

In addition to the above I set up a lunchtime rolling programme of board game activities (such as 'snakes and ladders') to be shared between two Year 6 children (who volunteered on a rota) and Suki, plus another girl (of Suki's choice) from Reception class.

During these board game sessions Suki did not feel under pressure because the focus of attention was drawn away from her, and directed onto the skill of participation in the game.

In this collaborative learning situation there was no unrelenting pressure being placed upon Suki, as nobody was asking her questions with the sole intention of coercing her to speak. In this non-threatening situation spoken words were not a requirement through which to participate.

Interestingly, after about six weeks two of the Year 6 girls came into my classroom at lunch-time. They looked very excited as they both walked quickly towards me. *Mrs Bligh, Mrs Bligh*, they called insistently. *What is it?*, I asked. In chorus they both said, *Suki's whispering!* As you can imagine I was thrilled. After many weeks of concern over Suki's lack of engagement in participation within the Reception class, I at last had a positive result – Suki was communicating alongside others in spoken English.

Approximately two weeks later, at 3.15pm Suki's mother collected her from class as usual at the end of the day. However, she returned to the classroom with Suki shortly afterwards and looked towards me with the intention of asking me a question. *Have you something you want to ask me?*, I gently queried. Suki's mother smiled at me and said *Suki has something to say to you Mrs Bligh*. Suki lifted her head and whispered in the softest of voices, *Goodbye Mrs Bligh*. This immensely uplifting moment was something that I will never forget.

Subsequently, little by little, Suki began to contribute in class. She never became a loud speaker, nor somebody who wished to be the centre of attention. And yet, at a pace set by herself, Suki's participation was increasing. She was fractionally increasing her participation in the practices of the early years setting. Within the non-pressurised environment of the Reception class, she felt able to turn her speech outwards through her additional language – English.

Critical questions

»   *How can teachers/practitioners mediate effectively in circumstances where they have no understanding of the child's cultural tools?*

»   *Is it possible to listen to the voices of emergent bilingual learners without sharing their mother tongue?*

»   *Is there another means of listening throughout the silent period?*

The research

This case study was drawn from a small part of an extended research inquiry (Bligh, 2011) that employed a multimethod ethnographic approach to data gathering, including participant observations of five key characters, unstructured interviews with monolingual participants, participant narratives and significant auto-ethnographic accounts. As part of a two-stage analytic process, data was funnelled through thematic analysis (Braun and Clarke, 2006) and tested out against sociocultural theorising.

The analysis reinforced Vygotsky's (1997a, b) thinking on children's learning processes, through which understandings of the social world are gained. It would appear that children do not learn in isolation, but act upon and adopt the ideas of others through appropriation (Rogoff, 1990) within their own participatory capacity. In line with the thinking of Vygotsky (1997a, b), Mehrotra et al. (2009) suggest that *the practices and tool use got transferred and embodied in other students' thoughts and practices* (Mehrotra et al., 2009, p 91). Although Bruner (1996, p 93) described an agentive mind as *proactive, problem-orientated, attentionally focused, selective, constructional and directed to ends*, the learning experiences of children like Suki conflict through everyday *practice at practice*, and they may feel *overwhelmed, overawed, and overworked* (Lave and Wenger, 1991, p 116) as their identity evolves in direct relation to their developing participatory practices.

The research findings

Through 'practising the practices' and increasing her participation in the social practices of the early years setting, Suki made these practices her own. However, learning through imitation differs from learning through guided participation (Rogoff, 2003), in that the modelling of practices within the early years setting appears to have been mainly incidental. Members of the early years community of practice were not necessarily modelling practices with the intent to mediate Suki's learning. However, Suki was actively and intentionally copying the practices of others.

Suki demonstrated such tensions through endless practice and engagement in participation, until eventually the 'inner workings' of the early years setting become 'part and parcel' of her own practices. The increasing levels of participation demonstrated by Suki were not just *a prelude to actual engagement* (Wenger, 1998, p 100); her practices enabled her to gain new understandings through fractionally increasing participation. Lave and Wenger's (1991) analysis confirms the importance of peripherality as an approximation of full participation in the provision of exposure to actual practice, thus encouraging 'newcomers' to move from peripheral to more central participation.

Vygotsky (1997a, b) was in no doubt that learning requires mastery and appropriation of signs and tools, with thought and language being the fundamental tools through which learning transforms the practices of the child. Suki's silent experiences confirmed the importance of thought as a fundamental tool for learning, and how children like Suki are capable of mediating their own learning (Drury, 2007, p 101). Vygotsky (1986, 1987) demonstrated that internalisation of Suki's spoken word (her mother tongue) resulted in a cognitive transformation (Vygotsky, 1978, p 86).

Interestingly, although Suki's spoken word appeared to turn inwards (became silent) it was not accompanied by the simultaneous unfolding of speech (Vygotsky, 1987). In fact, the development from thought to word was able to stop at any point, as was demonstrated through Suki's 'freezing' when she approached the school gates.

The research findings tentatively revealed that for an emergent young bilingual learner like Suki, the silent period presents as a phase of intense learning, through fractionally increasing participation. Drawing upon the sociocultural understandings of Lave and Wenger (1991) and Vygotsky (1978), it is evident that learning had taken place within and through participation with others.

Despite the demands put upon Suki, she nonetheless silently attempted to carve a ... *path to success in the face of the dominant monolingual discourse*. Gee and Green defined this agentive action as ... *changing patterns of participation in specific social practices within communities of practice* (1998, p 147).

The findings made apparent that through fractionally increasing participation:

* the emergent bilingual learner engages in silent participation on the periphery of practice;

* the silent period presents as a phase of intense learning, through fractionally increasing participation;

* the silenced mother tongue (as thought) acts as an agentive and self-mediating tool through which to participate and learn.

Pedagogical implications

The findings raise several interesting issues in relation to current early years pedagogy. The results would suggest that, in terms of current early years practice within the *Statutory Framework for the Early Years Foundation Stage* (DfE, 2012b), the provision of adequate quiet 'thinking' spaces within which a young bilingual learner can synthesise the practices of early years settings (digest her/his learning) is of crucial importance.

Notably absent in the findings is evidence of the early years teachers/practitioners *know-ingly* mediating learning during the silent period, and yet this mediatory role is crucial for learning (Vygotsky, 1978; Rogoff, 2003). Although not specifically designed to focus upon the silent period, Magraw and Dimmock's (2006) 'Merridale' nursery project revealed the important role of teachers in mediating children's peripheral participation through silence spaces.

> *We became aware of the length of silences during a session, when we listened to the audio recordings. On reflection we realised the inevitability of silences ... and that good relationships are based on the acceptance of them. We came to realise that presence is the other side of silence, and allows for the child to continue comfortably doing their self-allotted task, knowing that support and assistance is available if wanted, but it is not forced.*

(Magraw and Dimmock, 2006, p 4)

The teachers on the Merridale project guided the children's participation while allowing them to negotiate their own levels of participation through their silence. Each child's peripheral participation was legitimised by the teacher, who modelled practices that could be observed and copied without an expectation of dialogue.

Worthy initiatives such as the Coram Family project, 'Listening to Young Children' (Lancaster and Broadbent, 2003), have helped redefine the portrait of a child from that of passive to autonomous (Clark and Moss, 2001). However, such initiatives have been quickly super-seded by government-supported 'top-down' attempts to raise the status of 'speaking and listening' via the delivery of the 'Every Child a Talker' (ECAT) initiative (DCSF, 2008). However, in the process of attempting to raise the status of the spoken word, has the significance of the *unspoken* word been overlooked, both as a crucial cultural tool for bilingual learning? Although the government ECAT guidance (DCSF, 2008, p 9) states that *Modelling language and using descriptive commentary should make up about 80% of your interactions*, where is the acknowledgement of silence as a tool for learning? Would it not be possible to appreciate legitimate peripheral participation (LPP) within early years pedagogy as a 'workable' concept through which young bilingual learners might gain participation or a 'sense of belonging' within the early years setting?

Clark and Moss (2001) introduced the 'mosaic approach' as an appropriate methodological tool with which to hear the unspoken voices of children. The mosaic approach employs a range of observational tools to enable children to build up a 'mosaic' picture of their 'early years' experiences. For instance, a child might take a 'tour' of the early years environment (employing a camera as a research tool) to point out areas of interest, or draw a 'map' and/or pictures of 'things' they might dislike. This contemporary mode of thinking has raised questions not only regarding current UK attitudes towards the status of young children in terms of *empowerment* within early years learning environments, but also about the resourcefulness of children as *researchers* (Kellet, 2010). As a result of these incredibly enlightening studies, teachers/practitioners are encouraged to listen not only to the spoken, but also to the *unspoken* words, through *the hundred languages of children* (Rinaldi, 2005).

Early years teachers/practitioners are inevitably bound to government policy and practice through nationally introduced 'curriculums', such as the EYFS (DCSF, 2007). However, the nature of such frameworks is predominantly based upon developmental and cognitively based models of learning, as opposed to that of sociocultural theorising. Although of significance in early years practice, developmental and cognitively based models 'fall short' in not revealing the whole child.

Critical questions

» *Where is the acknowledgement of children's sociocultural history and learning outside school?*

» *Where is our acknowledgement of the international and cultural differences in the status of silence?*

The value of silence and the spoken word is unequally culturally distributed. In the western world, with speaking being aligned to higher-order assessments of cognitive development, contributions offered through silent participation go unrecognised. However, in countries such as Japan and India, silence and thoughtfulness (mother-tongue thinking) are highly valued. Trawick added that *silence in relationships in India does not mean absence but is more of a tool that invites dialogue, probing and further understanding* (1990, p 33). However, UK researchers such as Drury (2007) and Bligh (2011) reveal silence to be a powerful, assertive and agentive action.

INTERNATIONAL PERSPECTIVES

Set in India, Viruru's ethnographic nursery school study set out to question the high status bestowed solely upon the spoken word as the main vehicle of human expression and communication (Viruru, 2001; Viruru and Cannella, 2001). Interestingly, the study suggests that children *engage in complex forms of communication that do not involve language*, and therefore questions the common assumption in dominant western discourses that the spoken word should be monolingual when *most of the world's children use and live in multilingual environments*. Is this yet another example of the western world imposing its cultural norms upon less dominant cultures and communities – and in particular children? Viruru asks whose interests are best served when *[spoken] language is privileged over other modes of communication* (Viruru, 2001, p 31).

Based in a university in America, Kato's studies, which explore silence as participation (Kato, 2010) and cultures of learning (Kato, 2001), compare the learning of Japanese students with those of indigenous American students. Kato reveals that for *some Japanese students, silence is interpreted as a legitimate form of classroom participation* (2010, p 13). The Japanese students argued that non-verbal learning through such modes as *writing papers, taking notes during the class, listening to the teacher, and reading the assigned books* demonstrated alternative means of participating. However, although the students believed that silence was a legitimate means through which to participate in class, their teachers did not.

Without a culturally responsive pedagogy, not only does the cultural and linguistic diversity of the young children remain unacknowledged, but teacher–child interactions continue to be formulated solely through white, middle-class, monolingual and curriculum-formulated dictates, with the language of instruction projecting solely white, UK, middle-class cultural expectations – transferred (both verbally and non-verbally) through teachers'/practitioners' attitudes, values and expectations.

If bilingual learners are already disadvantaged by experiencing cultural discontinuity between home and school, then the knowledge base of the early years setting remains disconnected from the child's prior learning. There is little evidence that early years practitioners act as cultural brokers during the silent period, even though they are in the 'powerful' position of being able to 'make a difference' by actively drawing upon their funds of knowledge (Moll et al., 2005).

Although parents in the western world expect their children's lives to be full, active and stimulating (the spoken word considered as pivotal), it must be remembered that emergent bilingual learners participate through alternative and culturally appropriated means.

The hidden voice

Smith (2002) notes that within the evolving paradigm of 'childhood studies', psychological models of individual growth and development (independent of context) are currently being challenged (Woodhead, 2004), with a re-emphasis on the diversity of childhoods coming to the fore. According to Mayall (2004), instead of children being considered as 'mute', vulnerable objects of concern (Hardman, 1973), they are now repositioned as powerful and competent social actors with *voice* and *agency* – through agency children express their 'hidden' voice.

If a young bilingual learner gains participation through her/his silent experiences, then focusing predominantly on the spoken word may draw the child out of the 'security' of legitimate peripheral participation – thus hindering (or at worst blocking) the child's attempts to participate. The young child loses the 'look-out post' from which to participate silently.

Indeed, Hancock's study articulates how two-year-old children *use and invest meaning* in *safe* domestic spaces, through utilising their familiar signs, symbols and tools (Hancock and Gillen, 2007, p 1). Unfortunately, such spaces within which an emergent bilingual learner can silently make meaning (Bligh, 2011) are noticeable by their absence within English-speaking early years settings.

The findings would suggest that in terms of current early years practice, including the current EYFS (DCSF, 2007), the provision of adequate spaces ('look-out posts') through which a young bilingual learner can synthesise the practices within the early years setting might be considered crucial. Rogoff envisaged spaces where *learning activities are planned by children as well as adults, and where parents and teachers not only foster children's learning but also learn from their own involvement with children* (2000, p 3), thus developing understandings of how learning moves fluidly through and beyond the early years setting, into the wider community.

Critical questions

»   *Having read the case study, how has your thinking been challenged?*

»   *Are there areas within your practice that you would change in response to this case study?*

»   *Explain your reasons for the above.*

Further research

While raising significant and critical issues, this chapter identifies that there is much potential for several additional lines of inquiry to be pursued.

Firstly, the significance of the silent period (as a medium through which learning occurs) invites collaborative investigation. A comparative study of the silent period through contrasting theoretical lenses (cognitive-developmental and sociocultural) using both quantitative and qualitative methods within a larger cohort of participants might offer more substantive links between the findings and the wider population of emergent bilingual learners.

Future research into the silent period might benefit from investigating the less prominent (and yet significant) factors relating to 'feelings of isolation', and the 'affective' and 'cultural discontinuity'. Although this chapter has not attempted to address these issues, further qualitative inquiry might draw upon unseen and unsaid details. In addition, practitioners'/teachers' capabilities in addressing these significant 'sub-' factors and how they impact (or not) upon children's lived experiences within the silent period might invite future study.

The significance of silent spaces (Bligh, 2011) within the early years community is another focus of attention that invites sole (small-scale) as well as collaborative (larger-scale) research in relation to both the status of silence within current early years pedagogy and the value placed upon silence as a medium through which thinking and learning occur.

Examining the silent period through Suki's experiences raises several important issues – not only in relation to the diversity of meaning-making, but also the nature of our and others' understandings of ourselves. Indeed, Greene and Hill suggest that we should accept silence as our problem rather than the child's, when suggesting:

> *the nature of any child's experience is always in part inaccessible to an outsider ... This inaccessibility is even more problematic when children are as yet unable to report on their conscious encounters with the world ...*
>
> (Greene and Hill, 2005, p 5)

Young children like Suki need their alternative contributions to learning to be recognised and valued. In adding a unique, sociocultural perspective to current second-language-acquisition perspectives of bilingual learning, this chapter has succeeded in demonstrating silence as a means to provide the agency a young child requires to participate silently while legitimately situated in an early years setting – on the periphery of participation.

Summary

Akin to the children in Rose Drury's study of two sisters entering nursery provision (Drury, 1997), Suki entered an early years setting without the ability to mediate her learning through familiar and mutually shared cultural tools.

> *Children ... present a challenge to schools because their language use and their socialisation and cultural experience in and beyond the home, do not match the norm which teachers expect to be able to build on.*

(Drury, 1997)

Suki could not speak the dominant discourse because her mother tongue was not English; and without assisted mediation of her learning, a silent and unseen barrier developed between Suki, her teacher and participation with her peers. However, something happened that transformed Suki's meaning-making without any obvious support. Suki 'instinctively' sought out legitimate peripheral participation as a location through which to learn the practices of the early years setting – the Reception class. Without explicit guidance, Suki initially 'distanced' herself from the core practices of the early years setting, and while situated on the periphery of practice (legitimised by her monolingual peers) she began to learn. Through her mother-tongue thought processes Suki managed to engage in a rich mix of interconnected practices. Peering through a sociocultural lens, Suki's learning through participation could be realised.

Early years teachers and practitioners may currently be presented with limited colours (cognitive models) with which to articulate bilingual learning. Identifying that there are additional 'colours' available on the palette (applying a sociocultural perspective) may assist in developing further understandings of how best to support children like Suki through their 'monolingual' silent experiences, and into a familiar bilingual understanding.

Although this chapter makes apparent that the silent period is a critical time for negotiating the way into and through the early years setting, there remain three unanswered issues that need clarification.

Critical questions

» *Does sociocultural dissonance on transition into the school environment 'elongate' the silent period?*

» *Is the young additional language learner making an asserted choice of loyalty to the mother tongue by actively rejecting the majority language within the early years setting?*

» *How does a sociocultural perspective build upon the cognitively based second-language acquisition model?*

Observing Suki through a second-language-acquisition lens, it may appear that young bilingual learners like Suki employ non-verbal communication strategies solely as a prerequisite to English language learning. However, when viewed through a sociocultural lens these same 'strategies' are redefined as culturally appropriated practices through which to gain participation within the early years setting. Therefore, sociocultural theorising is seen to enhance cognitively focused models of second-language acquisition, through revealing new ways of knowing and meaning-making.

This chapter has not set out to offer 'top-down' *solutions* to the teaching of emergent bilingual learners. It does, however, emphasise the complexity of learning throughout the silent period, and reveals silent participation as a means through which an emergent bilingual learner 'practises the practices', and makes meaning within, through and beyond an early years setting. Applying a sociocultural perspective to an examination of the silent period tentatively reveals that, for emergent young bilingual learners, the silent period presents as a phase of intense learning, through fractionally increasing participation in the practices within the early years community.

During the silent period Suki's mother tongue appeared to turn inwards (as thought), and in doing so acted as an agentive and self-mediating tool through which she gained in participation – began to learn. To clarify: as the result of thought passing through *an infinite variety of movements; to and fro, in ways still unknown to us*, the agentive action of self-mediation *creates a connection, moves, grows and develops, fulfils a function, solves a problem* (Vygotsky, 1986, pp 254, 218).

Suki's case study also demonstrates that there is a preferred location for the emergent bilingual learner to gain knowledge of the early years practices. Legitimate peripheral participation offered Suki the ideal location (on the periphery of practice) through which to 'look in' on the early years practices. Through the 'look-out post' of legitimate peripheral participation Suki gained the ability fractionally to increase her participation.

Of critical concern is the finding that early years teachers/practitioners were less culturally responsive than might be expected in performing a mediatory role for emergent bilingual learners during the silent period (Deldado Gaitan, 2006). This is not to say that early years teachers and practitioners disregard the needs of additional language learners, but more that they are unsure (in the absence of guidance) as to what they should be doing during the silent period. In the absence of research-led, statutory guidance on the role of teacher-/practitioner-led mediation of (English Additional Language) learning within early years settings this is hardly surprising. Owing to the uncertainty of this mediatory role, and with much mediation being incidental, the young bilingual learner has been seen predominantly to mediate her/his own learning.

Parents in the western world may expect their children's lives to be full, active and stimulating, with the spoken word considered as pivotal. However, emergent bilingual learners participate through alternative and culturally appropriated means as demonstrated through the studies of Kato (2010, p 13), Trawick (1990) and Viruru (2001).

Suki's case study applied sociocultural learning theory as a means to 'unpack' the silent period. Historical understandings of Vygotsky (1986) provided a platform through which to examine Suki's silent experiences during her time spent in a Reception class setting.

Legitimate peripheral participation (Lave and Wenger, 1991) provided a workable concept through which to explore Suki's initial learning trajectory as she attempted to negotiate participation within, through and beyond the early years community of practice. Facilitating Suki's access to legitimate, peripheral participation assisted her in fractionally increasing her participation in the activities of the early years setting. Situated in a 'safe' location (on the periphery of practice) Suki was contributing to the shared learning.

Applying a sociocultural lens has been *less about revealing the external child and more about uncovering the historical child* (Fleer et al., 2004, p 175). Sociocultural understandings have revealed the complexity of Suki's learning within and throughout the silent period. Her silent experiences demonstrated that her learning did not follow a linear pathway, but moved across and through both the familiar and less familiar communities of practice of home and school (Wenger, 1998). Suki's self-mediated negotiation of practices served as her main means through which to gain new understandings of, and participation in, the unfamiliar world of the early years setting.

Providing a sociocultural perspective upon the silent period has revealed much about *how* Suki made meaning of her new world per se, as opposed to solely learning the language of spoken English. Although Suki's experiences inform us less about cognitive processing within the initial stage of English Additional Language learning, much more is revealed about the *practice* of learning throughout the silent period – whether it be learning how to be like the teacher, to be able to share in the practices of others or simply to 'fit in'.

Suki's case study contributes to our developing understandings of the role played by silent participation within a specific stage in additional-language acquisition – the silent period – demonstrating that sociocultural theorising aims to build upon second-language acquisition theory. One interpretation would be to say that a linguistic interpretation reveals part of a child's learning   that of language. However, with the additional layering of sociocultural theorising, the whole child is revealed – all of her/his practices within participation are made visible as one whole. This 'wholeness' surpasses the four walls of the early years classroom and permeates the interconnecting communities of both home and school.

Silence may still remain a misunderstood and undervalued phenomenon within UK culture, and yet through agentive and resourceful 'everyday' practices, the multicomplexity of the silent period is illuminated. The findings present learning through the silent period as fractional, complex and agentive. Young children like Suki need their alternative contributions to learning to be recognised and valued.

Struggling to fit in and belong is difficult at any time in a person's life, and for a young child like Suki it is even more so. Within the early years setting, the young bilingual learner may be unable to:

*   be understood when speaking in his/her mother tongue;
*   comprehend the language of instruction;
*   understand the nuances of spoken discourses.

However, even during this difficult period in an emergent bilingual learner's life-world the young child is capable of taking ownership of her/his own learning, both inside and outside the early years communities of practice. This resourcefulness in 'getting through' and in ultimately succeeding 'out there' in the multiplicity of the 'real world' is truly remarkable (Conteh, 2003). Therefore, silent, young bilingual learners are revealed as being capable of negotiating their own learning pathways during periods of intense uncertainty and are seen ultimately to succeed in doing so.

Critical reflections

Through your analysis of Suki's 'story', you should now be equipped to:

» *offer a sociocultural perspective on what is being experienced during the silent period;*

» *provide insight into learning through the silent period;*

» *explore the findings in relation to current early years pedagogy;*

» *relate Suki's experiences within the early years environment to the well-being of other young children in early years settings who encounter similar experiences.*

Further reading

The purpose of writing this chapter has been not only to engage the reader in critical thinking relating to a child's well-being within the silent period, but also to whet the reader's appetite to know more in relation to young bilingual learners' experiences in early years settings. The following suggested reading materials were chosen in part because of their significance in contributing to this field of study, and also because of their invaluable contributions in the evaluation of Suki's learning journey. I hope you enjoy reading them as much as I have.

Drury, R. (2007) *Young Bilingual Learners at Home and School: Researching Multilingual Voices.* Stoke-on-Trent: Trentham.

Rose Drury presents silence as a powerful and agentive action accessible to emergent bilingual learners who might otherwise appear as 'disempowered' in early years settings.

Flewitt, R. (2005) Is Every Child's Voice Heard? Researching the Different Ways 3-year-old Children Communicate and Make Meaning at Home and in a Preschool Playgroup. *Early Years: An International Journal of Research and Development*, 25(3): 207–22.

Rosie Flewitt demonstrates the multiplicity of non-spoken voices that young children employ within early years settings.

Magraw, I.; Dimmock, E. (2006) *Silence and Presence: How Adult Attitude Affects the Creativity of Children*. National Teacher Research Panel summary. Available from www.standards.dfes.gov.uk/ntrp/publications/. Accessed 26 July 2013.

Researched by practising early years teachers, this fascinating study provides extensive evidence of the importance of silence as a collaborative learning tool.

Lave, J.; Wenger, E. (1991) *Situated Learning: Legitimate Peripheral Participation*. Cambridge: Cambridge University Press.

Jean Lave and Etienne Wenger elucidate the significance of legitimate peripheral participation as a means to learning the practices within any given community of practice.

2 The parents' and extended family perspective

CHELLE DAVISON

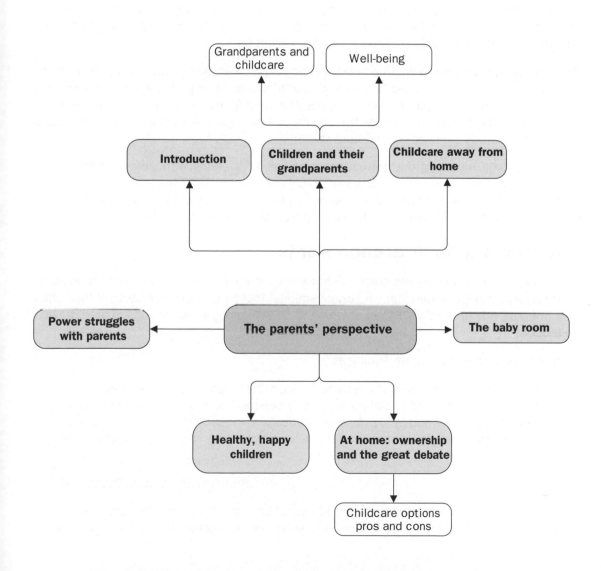

[P]arents' involvement during childhood is a predictor of educational attainment later in life. Thus time devoted by parents to Childcare is an important productive activity for society.

(Gioacchino, 2012)

Introduction

Despite the many guides and 'how to' books that line the shelves of the most well-known book shops, there still remains a vacant spot for the real guide to parenting. There might well be a book or magazine that claims to be the one and only real guide to parenting, but ultimately every reader will interpret each page, and each suggestion, in their own desperate way, hoping that this book will be the one to give them the golden words, the true real-life method of getting their toddler to sleep, or eat carrots, or throw away the dummy. Each parent or prospective parent scours the pages hoping for inspiration. Some may well find the answer they are looking for, most will throw it in the recycling believing they have already tried and tested the suggestions laid down in print, only to have found failure. Nothing seems to work with this particular child. Where is the rule book? Where is the comprehensive guide in which every suggestion works without fail? Who should that parent turn to?

This chapter will look at the various methods adopted by childcarers for working with parents and families to support children's learning, health and well-being. It will offer case studies that span the breadth of parental experiences, the need for quality childcare, and the differences between a parent's desire for the healthy well-being of their children and the institutionalised methods of childcare and education.

Why are we still repeating the normalised practices of 'working with parents'? Perhaps it is because we have failed to see how such practices are contradicting the desires of those same parents and their children. We know every family works in a different way, so do professionals reflect this difference in how they support children's well-being?

Children and their grandparents

When you start a search for the definition of well-being, the search engine takes you to many child-protection papers, websites and organisations. To a parent, the well-being of their child may not instantly or readily suggest anything to do with the general notions related to child protection.

Statham and Chase defined well-being as:

> *the quality of people's lives. It is a dynamic state that is enhanced when people can fulfil their personal and social goals. It is understood both in relation to objective measures, such as household income, educational resources and health status; and subjective indicators such as happiness, perceptions of quality of life and life satisfaction.*

(Statham and Chase, 2010, p 2)

A parent is concerned with the happiness of their child, their health and, in most cases, their education. To a parent their child's happiness is far from subjective. It has to be guaranteed.

It is not enough for a childminder to say *Oh, I think they had fun today*. However, when a grandparent recounts their trip to a supermarket, the bank and the market, the parent may willingly accept this seemingly mundane experience for the child, discounting the possible reduction in fun and learning. There is something ironic in a parent's decision where to place their child while they are at work. On the one hand a parent has the highest expectations from a setting that they pay for, wanting high-quality care, a strong learning environment and behavioural training. On the other, some parents choose grandparents, who are most often working on a voluntary basis and fit the childcare into their own busy lives, choosing to take the child or children along to the more routine visits; supermarkets, corner shops and banks. A grandparent may part with the information that the child has slept for two hours, or has been changed throughout the day, but they are very unlikely to explain how many sounds the child has mastered or their understanding of 'more or less'. It is strange to me that paid childcare is required to educate and instruct a child, while a grandparent need only babysit.

In September 2008, the UK government introduced and implemented the new early years curriculum: Early Years Foundation Stage (EYFS). A curriculum that is complex and challenging but one that is statutory nonetheless. Yet thousands of preschool children are cared for by family and friends in informal agreements made by parents looking either for a cheaper option or, as in many cases, for a more homely, less formal environment.

Grandparents and childcare

Very little research has been done so far on the impact that grandparents have on the well-being of the children they care for. The concept is overshadowed by a variety of other debates such as mothers in employment, moving single parents back into employment and, more recently, the quality of childcare and ratios debate (Nutbrown, 2013; BBC, 2013; Channel 4, 2013).

Parents are a complicated group within society, and much has changed since the stay-at-home mum was the norm, with an increase in divorce, in single parents, and in families deviating from what we know as the 'nuclear' family to favour same-sex parents and parents cohabiting while unmarried. Netmums published a survey where they claimed to have results showing more than 35 different types of family residing in the UK (Netmums, 2013). The survey showed that more than 20 per cent of families were led by unmarried parents and 10 per cent by single parents, while more than 6 per cent were blended families where there were a mix of biologically related family members and stepfamily members living together. This is no longer a shock to parents generally; according to the US Census Bureau, Statistical Abstract of the United States: 2012, the percentage of births to single women in the UK went up from 11.5 per cent in 1980 to 43.7 per cent in 2006. In addition to all of the differing family units, these in turn make extended family units more complex, with some children engaging with three or even four sets of grandparents (Sanders and Trygstad, 1989).

Meyers and Swiebert (1999, p 1) suggest that there is a new but nonetheless important need for specific counselling and support aimed at a new breed of grandparents: those that have resulted from the divorce and remarriage of their children. Relationships are crucial to the healthy development of a child, and the relationship with the child's grandparents, according to Meyers and Swiebert, is critical:

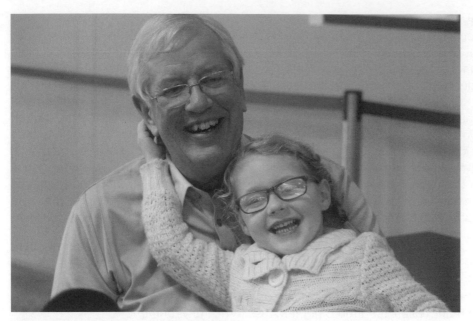

Figure 4 Grandfather and granddaughter

> *[C]hildren benefit from relationships with their grandparents affectively, cognitively and materially. They also give much to the relationship, including joy, inspiration, love, tenderness, closeness, companionship and hope for the future.*
>
> (Kalliopuska (1994), cited in Meyers and Swiebert (1999))

CASE STUDY

I would prefer all my children had been with their grandparents instead of a variety of childcarers. They go and spend the weekend and come home raving about their trips to the zoo or the cinema; they go walking through the woods and along canal sides. I remember the first time my little girl pointed out matter-of-factly that she had seen a butterfly and that the bird on our fence was a jackdaw. I thought I was the only one interested in the natural world. We ended up listening for bird song and pointing out which type of bird had been making their call. If I had to choose a time, just one, where I knew without doubt they were all completely carefree and entirely happy, I'd say it was when they stay with their grandparents.

(Vicki, 32)

Well, I get to go the cinema and they give us treats and things. We get to, like, sleep in in the mornings and we stay up quite late. We have supper with them (with sugar on) and we get to buy sweets and toys. We get to go to some castles and museums and they have loads of books to read. Granddad is quite cool – he scares my sisters when he takes out his teeth. He likes watching car-racing. Granny is fun and likes to do jigsaws and card games with us. Granny takes us loads of places. Granny's food is awesome; tea is always nice.

(Francis, 9)

Sarti (2010) discusses the Italian model where the working parent often chooses informal childcare with grandparents. Despite the earnings of the parents far exceeding that needed for paid childcare, the preference is to use grandparents. In 1998 only 6 per cent of Italy's babies attended a nursery paid for by their parents – the lowest percentage of any European country at that time – and by 2009 that figure had grown by only a further 3 per cent. Sarti also contends that over 79 per cent of the babies who occupied a nursery place had mothers who were in employment, arguing that mothers in employment *have a higher need to have help* (Sarti, 2010, p 795).

> *Grandparents ... play a crucial role in child raising ... in 1998 43.7% of children under the age of three and 42.8% of those between three and five, including those who went to day nurseries and nursery schools, were looked after by grandparents*
> (Sarti, 2010, p 796)

Well-being

In the UK, numerous organisations who champion grandparents acknowledge that the well-being of children is improved when they have a secure relationship with their grandparents:

> *Older people are ... important and valued member[s] of their family and these relationships need to be sustained. Such connections are central to an older person's wellbeing and to that of their children, friends and relatives.*
> (Smethers, 2010, p 396)

Smethers goes on to posit that grandparents are essential to the economic success of society and that the input that they have is an undervalued resource. As life expectancies continue to increase, children become grandparents who contribute to the upbringing of the children financially and educationally, and remain in good health long enough to see great-grandchildren come into their world.

Certainly you need only to walk into a coffee shop or take a stroll through the local market on a week day to see dozens of grandparents pushing buggies and negotiating a world that is so very distant from the world in which they brought up their own children. Nonetheless, grandmothers can be seen meeting other grandmothers, all settling into the routines of bank visits, coffee-shop breaks and nappy changes. Is that all we can see?

On one of my own visits to the town centre I watched a grandparent explain to a toddler why they could hear their own voice repeating over and over after they had shouted while in the confined area of a market entrance:

> *[Child shouts]*
> *Grandparent:* Can you hear your voice?
> *[Child repeats noise]*
> *Grandparent:* That is called an echo; your voice is bouncing off those walls.
> *[Child repeats noise]*

It occurred to me that even the most routine activities, the trips grandparents must make, provide invaluable learning for the children they care for, be it about a bird call, a leaf, a new insect or the echoes inside a market entrance. Grandparents may well be the financial answer for working mothers, but they are also the children's teachers: teachers who do not

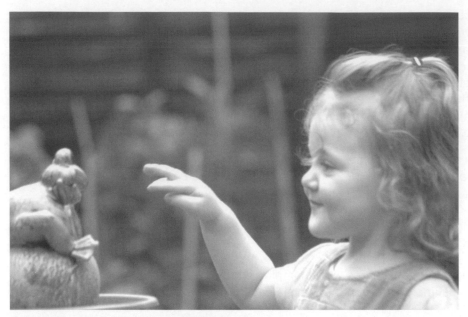

Figure 5   Nanna's garden wonderland

request payment or training for a new curriculum; teachers who cherish the five-minute lessons on sounds and echoes without having to write them in a learning journey or on a 'What I did today' form; teachers who have already successfully educated one generation without the EYFS curriculum as guidance to their children's development.

CASE STUDY

One of my children is more sensitive than the others. She's what I would call emotionally immature. She excels in school and loves nothing more than reading an entire Dr Seuss book to me out loud. Still, she's quiet, keeps close to one friend rather than a class full; I feel like I need to be more careful about the people that take care of her. I think she reminds me of myself when I was six. I was always told not to stare at people, to talk to them, say hi and goodbye. My parents' friends made me feel different and abnormal; I just didn't trust adults immediately like some children do – I watched how they behaved and how they spoke. I evaluated for myself whom to trust, but because I didn't race through the world like a 'normal' child, adults treated me as though there was a problem with me. My little girl reminds me of that time and maybe I do go a little overboard to protect her well-being, but I never want her to feel different, or that her way of evaluating her world is wrong. So I'm really careful whom she stays with for long periods of time. I eliminate anyone who questions her shyness or tries to label her observing as something negative. The only place other than home that I ever feel completely happy for her to go is to her grandparents. They treat her like she's perfect, and she is.

(Vicki, 32)

In 2012, Wellard estimated the worth of the informal childcare provision by grandparents to be in the region of £3.9 billion (Wellard, 2012), so why do some parents choose informal childcare – more specifically, grandparents?

*[D]espite the greater availability and affordability of formal early childhood educa-
tion and childcare, the number of parents using informal childcare – from friends
and family – remains nearly as high as formal childcare usage. Yet there is very
little knowledge about why parents make these childcare choices, about who provides informal childcare and about the impact of non-parental informal childcare
on children.*

(Daycare Trust, 2011)

Childcare away from home

For those parents who choose to use paid childcare outside the home, it can be a daunt-
ing task to find a setting where quality seems high and other parents speak highly of it.
In some cases parents arrive knowledgeable of early years and experienced in the art of
communicating their wishes to the staff involved. In other cases knowledge is severely
lacking and they rely on the staff in the setting to explain how things work, how things
are organised and what to expect. What remains astonishing is that parents will view a
house a number of times before buying it, will research the area, maybe even look to see
what the crime level is or where the 'good' schools are located. However, when it comes to
choosing childcare – a setting where their child may reside for up to 12 hours or more each
day – a parent seems happy with one or two visits and one or two 'settling-in' sessions. A
setting can be chosen after experiencing the staff and the environment for less than one
working day.

The Daycare Trust offers help to parents choosing childcare; they suggest using the Family
Information Service (FIS) locally, then visiting a number of settings, before finally, on their
third step only, they suggest parents *make the big decision* (Daycare Trust, 2011). Parents
who are aware of Ofsted can use the guidance on the Ofsted Website in their search for childcare, which suggests looking at the history of a setting, or they can view the Ofsted report
published for every Ofsted-registered setting (Ofsted, 2013).

When speaking with parents, a practitioner must understand that the level of knowledge a
parent has differs from family to family. Consider a mother delivering her child into the hands
of a Level 3-qualified member of staff. That member of staff will have a profoundly different
impact on the child and on their mother, primarily because of the expectations the mother
has in the first place; everything is dependent on what 'Mum' already understands about
early childhood care and learning. Another example is that of a mother who is trained in early
childhood education, and who may well feel excluded, purposely ignored or decisively cut out
from the world her child is about to enter because staff are worried as to how they will successfully converse with a knowledgeable parent.

Equally, the nervous parent who has no experience of children or childcare may feel overwhelmed and out of their depth, causing them to 'stop, drop and go'. No matter the background of a family, a professional must find the correct balance of 'conversation and
questioning' that suits the parent, the child and the setting.

Critical questions

» Reflect upon the last time you opened the door to a parent. What did you say? How did you feel?

» Consider how the parent may have felt leaving their child at that time. Was what you said equitable to the fact that their most important possession was about to be left in your hands? Would the parent feel confident and trusting, or happy to be leaving? Could you have done anything better?

CASE STUDY

The reality of appropriate childcare

I recall a conversation I had with a relatively new online organisation that had developed a system whereby parents could leave feedback on their experiences of a childcare setting. So I could log onto their web pages, type in the Ofsted reference numbers or the name of the setting, and leave a rating and additional comments if I chose to. I thought it would be a good idea – as a parent, the people I listened to most were other parents. They know a good setting, they listen to their children. So I began the task of giving feedback on all the settings I had previously used, as well as the ones I was still using. About three days later I received a load of e-mails telling me that the organisation didn't believe my feedback and asking if I could prove that I used the settings as a parent. I was astonished. They were basically telling me that I was lying. Instead of e-mailing back, I telephoned them.

Their response amazed me more than the e-mails. I was clearly told that no parent could possibly use all of the settings I had left feedback for.

I explained very clearly, slowly and with obvious irritation that I have four children. My eldest I placed in two Nurseries. The first I removed him after a week when I picked him up spotlessly clean and not having moved from the spotless carpet I had placed him on at 8am that morning. The second I loved; he had permanent access to the outdoors in a small, purpose-built bungalow where they followed my 'no routine, let him decide' policy. He slept when and where he chose, and ate when and where he chose. I was studying at university, with one child; he stayed only a few hours a week and I paid a fortune for the flexibility to drop him off and pick him up as and when I chose.

Then we moved house. I made more mistakes. We chose a brand new nursery: new building, new equipment, new staff and new management. It looked good inside and out. The outdoor area was amazing even by my standard. Within six weeks our bright, bubbly, confident little boy had disappeared. Every time I asked him about playing outside he would turn away from me and say 'Not been out today.' The decision to remove him from a second poor-quality setting came about when I drove down the road on which the setting was located and he started yelling 'Not rainbow house, not rainbow house.' That wasn't the setting's name, but for my two-year-old the logo had been imprinted into his mind and he told me in no uncertain terms he wasn't happy going there; the shiny new furniture and engaging management weren't enough for this little boy. So, we lost our deposit and a month's fees and I took a week off work to find better childcare.

Our next choice might surprise the more experienced of you. I took a parent's recommendation over the satisfactory Ofsted report and booked an appointment to see the *manager. Recounting the experiences we'd had over the last few weeks, I pointed out that we'd lost the trust of our two-year-old; he didn't believe we would leave him somewhere fun, or safe or loving, where he could thrive and develop just as if he were at home. Within another four weeks, and with the support of a family-friendly manager and a level 3-qualified room leader, our little boy's smile was back. It didn't make me feel better for having chosen a poor setting twice in his short 24 months under our care. He yelled every metre of the drive from where the old setting was until we passed it by and reached the new, less shiny setting: a reminder every morning that his parents had got it wrong.*

When my second child was about to come into the world, I was absolutely sure an external childcare setting was not my preferred choice for either child. I searched high and low for a nanny to allow them both to stay in their own home, to dictate their own routine and decide how their day was to be planned. I interviewed for almost my entire pregnancy using some of the most highly rated nanny agencies across the north. I couldn't find anyone.

The most significant meeting – and the shortest – was when a 40-plus lady arrived on my doorstep, introducing herself and towering over me, making me feel like I'd stepped back into grammar school and had a meeting in the head teacher's office. As she sat down I recounted her CV, which stated she had indeed been a school teacher. As I began the usual conversation by explaining that we had no set routine for our children, I nearly laughed out loud as her face crumpled into a confused frown and she repeated 'No routine, no routine?'. With an about-turn she promptly stood up and left. Without any further conversation.

The nanny we did find was through our own advertising in the local newspapers: a Level 3-qualified young girl who didn't fancy the confines of a nursery setting. We watched her negotiate our three-year-old and a new-born out of our back door and into the nearby park. I remember the smell of the wet leaves and the brisk February breeze as she pushed our little boy on the swing and carefully eyed the pram with our tiny pink bundle inside. She was hired. We left the decision to our eldest, and at not quite three years old he chose better childcare than his parents had, with all their experience and training.

(Caroline, 33)

The baby room

Many researchers have concluded what those with any experience of babies already know: children are born ready. Ready to explore, ready to see, ready to taste and touch and feel. They are more than ready to learn about the world around them (Gopnik et al., 1999; Greenfield, 2000; Meltzoff and Prinz, 2002). We are lucky to be able to pick up ongoing research that tells us very clearly how the important interactions and relationships that babies experience during their first days and months serve to provide distinct patterns of behaviour later in their developmental life, but they are not empty vials that will be filled with emotional experiences – they are interactive, capable individuals who exact their own interpretation of those around them. They relate in their own way.

Relatedness is in itself intersubjective and we have seen different babies elicit different responses in the same carers. Babies both shape and are shaped by the world of relationships into which they emerge.

(Gerhardt, 2006, p 305)

Without doubt, one of the hardest days of a mother's life will be the day she returns to work: the return to a career that she knows she must maintain for financial reasons, or maybe for aspirational reasons. Whatever the motive, leaving her tiny baby behind moves against every fibre of her being, and every feeling she has so carefully developed over the course of her pregnancy and delivery (see Figure 6). Nonetheless, that mother will, along with thousands of other women, walk out of the door leaving her baby in another's, trusted, hands.

Critical questions

»   *Do mothers understand with whom they are leaving their children?*

»   *When was the last time you shared with a parent your skills, knowledge or qualifications?*

Research as far back as the 1900s shows clearly that the majority of carers in childcare settings are young women who are not necessarily mothers themselves. There is no question that a person can care effectively for a child or baby without having children themselves; nonetheless, it could be argued that these young girls struggle to understand and empathise with the separation anxiety felt by both the child and the mother. That being said, empathy is not only an inherent skill but is also a learnt skill, and as a professional gains confidence and experience so their ability to understand separation anxiety, in both adult and child, grows. Ensuring that a mother, or father, is confident to leave their child in a setting outside the family is essential to a professional in being able to contribute to the formation of a secure, independent child. Harrison and Ungerer (2002, p 758) state that *Mothers who expressed more commitment to work and less anxiety about using non-family child care, and who returned to work earlier, were more likely to have secure infants.* Confident mothers (and fathers) can lead to confident babies.

Babies move through a variety of stages marked by their attachment to significant carers, parents and family. At around 18 months a child's fear of strangers is at an all-time high, as they determine who, apart from their primary attachment, is safe. With the family-friendly policies implemented by government, the possibility of extended maternity leave means that babies can be placed in childcare from the age of three months onwards, and significantly from 12 to 18 months, just as they begin to understand that there are other adults in the world.

Research into the smooth transition from a child's home – and therefore the primary carer – to formal, non-family childcare, has been significant, both in the past and in the present. Trying to develop new practice and refine older routines to ensure that the very best and most up-to-date methods of transition are implemented on a daily basis has meant that research into these early transitions has been immense (Blatchford et al., 1982; Wittenberg, 2001; Greenfield, 2011).

Greenfield (2011, p 100) highlighted *tensions* between parents and schools during the transition from home or childcare. I would argue that these tensions are not limited to schools but also occur during the transition from home to other formal childcare. A parent places ultimate trust in the expertise of the childcarer; they believe that carer is the best person for the care and education of their child. Be it a teacher, an educator, a level 3, a level 2, a manager, a deputy, an early years professional (EYP) or an early years teacher (EYT): whatever their title, whatever their name, a parent trusts that the person caring for their child while they are absent will care for them as if they were their own.

CASE STUDY

Does day care damage your baby? One mother's view ...

Having packed off three babies to nursery, I couldn't do it to my fourth baby.

When my first child Raymond was just over four months old, I put him in a day nursery. I was working part-time and used a nearby nursery from 8am to 6pm. When I visited, it all looked great. The staff were friendly. The lady who ran it seemed very committed to the children. I was told where Raymond would sleep during the day, what he would eat. I went to talk to the girl who headed up the baby room. Her name was Gemma and she was very young, but she came across as being capable and likeable. 'We get them in a routine here', she told me confidently.

On the first day, when I dropped him off, baby Raymond screamed his head off. 'Oh, don't worry', said Gemma, taking him from me, 'he'll get used to it'. Except he didn't. Every time I dropped him off, he would pummel his little feet against me and cling and scream. As Gemma took him, he would give me such a desperately panicked look, it would make me want to turn around and spirit the two of us back home again.

'Is this normal?', I asked. 'Oh, yes', said Gemma, firmly prising Raymond from my grasp. 'He'll adjust. They all do.'

By the fourth week, he had adjusted somewhat, so I convinced myself that Raymond was enjoying nursery. Still, I had misgivings. I felt guilty that he wasn't getting the one-to-one attention I felt he deserved. I was concerned about the regulation cots lined up against the wall, but reasoned it was the best option I had. After all, thousands of women drop their babies and preschoolers off at nurseries every day. How bad could it be?

Then, one day, I went to pick Raymond up early. I turned up at the nursery and, looking through the window, saw Raymond standing in his cot, absolutely sobbing. His face had gone red. I waited for someone to go and comfort him, but no one moved a muscle. All the staff were in the corner taking no notice. He wasn't the only baby crying. Four more were bellowing their heads off. I stormed into the room, picked Raymond up and asked Gemma what on earth she and her staff thought they were doing.

'It's their quiet time', she explained. 'We don't pick them up during quiet time.'

'He was crying', I said. 'He needs cuddling.' She said that the nursery had rules and regulations. 'I'm sorry', she said, 'but that's how we get the children to adjust'.

This is the problem with nursery care; one size has to fit all. Staff have to stick to a routine in order to survive day-in, day-out with a rotating set of children. The trouble is, children don't work this way. They are all different, with their different characteristics and needs. What I witnessed is something I have heard from other parents time and time again. Essentially, many feel let down by the quality of care and the lack of real affection shown to their children by day-care staff.

Still, I tried again, at a different centre, with my next two children, both boys – but they also hated it. My older boy complained the carers did nothing with him; the younger refused to eat any food that was cooked for him. Every time I dropped them off, they would both cry. I would stand there with two wailing children attached to my legs. The day they point-blank refused to get out of the car, I gave up.

By the time it came to my fourth and last child, my daughter, Sparkle, I didn't bother with nursery. All she has ever done is go to a local playgroup for a few mornings a week.

Now she's at school, and her teacher is amazed she never went to nursery. 'She's coping so well', she says. 'She's so happy and confident.' For me, that's the upside of not sending her to day care.

I do understand that, for many parents, day care is the only option. Without any close relations living nearby, and not being married to a house-husband, I also felt that way. But I am now fortunate not to have to send my children to nursery, and for that I am extremely grateful.

(Cavendish, 2011 © Telegraph Media Group Limited, 2011)

Critical questions

» *Consider parents who leave their children with you, in school, in day-care or another setting. Would you know how a parent feels about leaving their child? Do you know if they would prefer another option?*

» *Critically reflect upon the routines you are asked to follow. Are they based in research, theory and tested methodology, or are they routines preferred by staff/ management?*

At home: ownership and the great debate

There is something special about the familiarity a child feels when they are exploring in their own home. As a child takes their first steps and negotiates the outdoors; as a child looks carefully upon the flowers, the grass, the sky; they determine for themselves where is safe, what they can touch and how they decide to move forward.

The debate rages, even as we write these words, as to the best place for a child to be raised: at home, at school, in a nursery or with a childminder. The preferences of parents are not only fickle but they are often made out of pressurised necessity rather than from a well-planned and thought-out set of actions. Word of mouth from trusted colleagues, peers or toddler-group mums can often be more important than the Ofsted grading of *Good* or *Outstanding* – assuming a parent even knows what Ofsted means and how to access their reports.

So how does a parent decide where their child goes to at the point that they have to return to work? If headlines are to be believed, the contradiction and conflict over where or with whom to place their child can descend into utter chaos, thus raising the stress levels of a decision that ultimately has to be made, and is exclusively the parent's own.

The simple question of whether full-time nursery care for under-twos is good or bad for the child is not simple in the least. Academics and childcare experts not only disagree on the answer, but also on whether we have enough evidence to be equipped even to hazard an answer.

(Gentleman, 2010)

Consider the following two scenarios.

CASE STUDY

The toddler at home

B woke up this morning about 8am, I think. I'm not really sure – she had breakfast and then I took the others to school. We played outside for a little while and then I went and put some washing in. I made jam sandwiches for lunch. I picked up the children from school about 3.15.

(Observation made of B, 8.30am)

B empties out her drawers until she finds the pink jeans she is looking for, and the red, long-sleeved top she layers with a sun dress. The red top is inside out and the pink sun dress back to front. As she carefully negotiates the stairs (because her jeans come below her toes) she wanders into the dining room and climbs up onto 'her' chair to eat the cereal that has already been placed into her bowl. After watching the business of her siblings getting ready for school, she says 'bye' to each one as they go out of the front door. Still chewing her cereal, which she now has in her hands, she goes out of the back door and plays with her dog. Confidently, she wraps her arms around the dog's neck and they both roll to the floor. B gets back up to her feet and runs into the house without stopping. She runs into her parents' room: 'Daddy's not here, he's gone to take my sisters.'

(10.30am)

B has been playing happily by herself outside. She wanders between each of the growing plants to smell them: 'Mmm, nice, mmmm, nice.' She smells a mint bush and moves to some seedlings: 'Mmm, peas – you can't eat them, you're a dog.' Picking up a tub of coloured chalks, B begins making straight lines and circles on the paving stones. Her drawings begin to take the shape of the story she is telling: 'My sister's gone to school; my Dad's in the cellar; my dog can't eat the peas...' (see Figure 6)

(12.30pm)

With a sandwich in hand, B collects two books from the side of a cabinet in the dining room. She returns to the table and begins opening and closing the covers, turning two pages and changing the books. B gets up from her chair and moves towards a closed drawer across the room; she stands up on tiptoe so that she can reach into the drawer and remove a handful of coloured pencils and pens.

She returns to the table and sits quietly, colouring the pictures in the two books, and drawing more lines and circles.

(2.30pm)

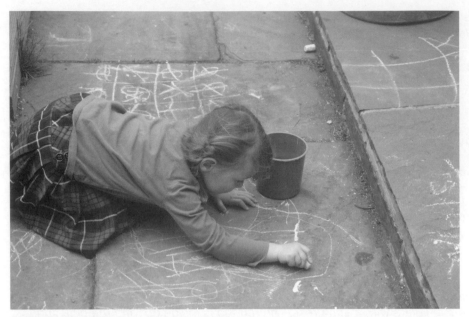

Figure 6 'B' drawing on the paving stones

Spinning around while holding a phone, B says that she is 'dancing for the phone fairies'.

CASE STUDY

The toddler in nursery

Between 8 and 9 we all have breakfast. Then they can go and play with whatever they want to, or they can do the activities that we set up on the tables. There's always an adult on the tables. Lunch is at 11.30 and we clear everything away before one of the staff brings out the plastic bowls and cutlery. Then they can go away and play again; if it's nice outside we go out to play but there is a rota so that everyone isn't outside at the same time. Snack is at around 3 and a light tea at 4.30. We usually ask parents to give them a proper tea at home.

(Observation made of A, 8.30am)

A arrived at about 8.35am, and Mum passed him to a member of staff (key worker's day off). The staff member put A into a high chair with six other babies lined up in a row. Two babies were being fed, one was asleep, and baby A sat quietly without food or activities. Mum stated 'he's already had breakfast', and left. A remained in the high chair with no food or activity for 25 minutes until breakfast time was over.

(11.00am)

All the babies and toddlers were allowed access to any toys on the floor. A picked up a ball and threw it into a dark tent. The ball lit up as it rolled into the tent. A picked up a wooden block and threw it into the dark tent, saying 'It's dark.'

(5.45pm)

A began falling asleep on the bean bag that was placed against the wall. A member of staff picked A up and stood him on his feet saying 'No sleeping, A, Mummy is here soon.' A sleepily wandered over to a group of children playing with cars. He looked across to the member of staff, seemingly to gain permission to play. Once the member of staff had nodded to him, he walked back to the bean bag and put the car into his pocket. The member of staff stood up and announced that it was home time and that children should 'come along and get your coats on ready'.

I haven't included the most extreme examples of home-care and care in a setting. Sometimes it can be difficult to dissect the two available options for parents and ensure that they are making a decision for their child, and that parents are confident they have chosen well.

Based on my own extensive experiences, it is my belief that children under the age of two should not be in a formal environment; however, there is certainly a considerable assortment of research that suggests babies do very well in formal childcare settings. Indeed, even the coalition government argues that very young children will benefit from *good-quality childcare*.

That said, it is difficult to see how a baby can benefit from being sat in a high chair with no food and no activity, simply because the other children are eating and because it is 'how we do things'. Placing eight babies into high chairs is certainly a method of control, but who is considering what those children are missing out on while they are being herded, and are restrained by plastic chairs?

The case study above highlights how difficult it really is to manage the logistics of family and carer. I have walked into nursery settings where babies are screaming through a monitor that is being ignored by professionals the other side of the room. So much needs to be altered in the repetitive routines of early years professionals.

One cannot ignore the fact that freedom of play, the opportunity to choose for themselves and the support children have to gain the confidence to learn are all part of being at home. Assuming they are given access to resources, time and spaces, children can learn and develop effectively while remaining at home prior to attending school. It is accepted that some children do not have the same opportunities and do not have the same access to resources as their counterparts; however, parents who value education, development and learning can and do provide learning experiences wherever possible. Parents do want the very best for the well-being of their children.

Once a child is handed over to formal childcare, those relaxed learning experiences are interrupted. That is not to say that settings cannot provide a comfortable environment – they can. However, it is my belief that before a child is two years of age they are less able to communicate exactly what they prefer. To stay at home or not to stay at home? The parent can be extraordinarily isolated from knowledge of exactly what is happening within a setting on a daily basis.

At home a child can explore, run, jump, eat and sleep whenever they choose. Routines are in place inside nurseries and schools because routine supports adult control over a group of young children, sometimes much like a military operation. Why do professionals march their children inside when it rains?

Table 2 Comparing childcare options: pros and cons

Home-care positives	Home-care negatives
Child has freedom of entire house; no routine	Adults miss opportunity to extend learning
Activities are chosen by child	Learning to use a tool may be missed
Activities are stopped/started by child	Adult scaffolding is unavailable
Development of all EYFS areas	Assessment of skills may be missed
Sleep is chosen by child	
Food is chosen by child	Food is chosen and prepared by adult
Resources are available throughout	Resources may not be age-appropriate
Setting/school-care positives	**Setting/school-care negatives**
Child has a routined day where things happen regularly	A set routine for each day restricts the activities a child can do
Activities are chosen by child and adults	Activities can be adult-led for parents, learning journeys and displays
Some activities are started/finished by the child	Children are required to participate in scheduled activities
Development of all EYFS areas	Assessment against a standardised curriculum using averages, rather than individual attainment and development
Resources are plentiful	Resources are restricted by adults
Food is nutritious	Times for eating are dictated by adults; choice of foods is determined by adults
Access to outdoors available	Time is on a rota system; access to outdoors during winter months is often restricted

The range of options for parents is not always clear. Parents believe that settings must be good places for children because otherwise they would be closed – wouldn't they? Childminders who can pass an Ofsted inspection without a paediatric first aid certificate, without having undergone any EYFS training and with children having access only to a wide-screen TV – they don't exist, do they? Parents tend to trust the people around them who are going through similar experiences, such as friends and colleagues who recommend a nursery, a childminder or a nanny.

The cost of childcare has recently been a huge topic of discussion in the early years sector and within government. Every corner, every element that plays a part in early years care and education is offering an opinion. In the frenzy that is the world around our children, how are parents represented?

Hiring a nanny to care for more than one child at home is significantly less costly than placing more than one child into nursery. A childminder may be cheaper than a nanny, but the children are ultimately in someone else's home, and are restricted by the regulations of Ofsted and registration.

Critical questions

» *There has been an explosion of childcare settings (various) over the past 20 years. Many are only partly filled, many have vacancies. Is it possible to retain choice for parents, reduce settings in number and impact the cost for parents?*

» *Critically evaluate the process of choice for parents. How do you play a part in that choice?*

» *Critically reflect on your training and experience. How do you ensure 'quality' is the key focus of your practice?*

Healthy, happy children

For most parents the good health of their children is paramount. Parents want to see their children running free, happy, healthy and thriving. It is arguably an innate characteristic of becoming a parent, and for many women and some men the instinctive desire begins the day they find out they will become parents. That being said, governments across the world spend millions on campaigns encouraging parents to take better care of their children's teeth and weight and to have their children immunised against various childhood diseases (Arrow et al., 2013; Hand et al., 2013).

How much parents trust the expertise of professionals is a subject that has already been touched upon, and is of importance when parents choose (or don't choose) to engage with other professionals in the care and education of their children. Are we trusted as professionals and, conversely, are we trusted as parents?

Unfortunately professionals are often mere puppets in the hands of government. As the government changes its policy, as organisations such as the World Health Organization (WHO) make changes to their policies, so professionals on the front line change their practices. Rightly or wrongly, change occurs in accordance with a higher power. If the professionals themselves do not question these changes, if the professionals themselves toe the line without any challenge or personal research, so parents will follow – assuming they trust the professional in front of them.

Even the professionals themselves end up confused over what they should or should not be advising parents. Take breastfeeding as an example. In 2002 the WHO published its report *The Optimal Duration of Exclusive Breastfeeding: A Systematic Review* (Kakuma, 2002), in which it advised that there were *no apparent risks in recommending as a general policy exclusive breastfeeding for the first 6 months of life* (p 20). Later, in 2011, a study published by the *British Medical Journal* (Fewtrell et al., 2011) suggested that weaning a baby, or introducing solid foods alongside breast milk, might actually reduce allergies later in the child's development. As you might imagine, the contradiction between exclusive breastfeeding until six months and weaning as early as four months meant that some mothers were left completely confused and even less trusting of advice given to them by health visitors and other such professionals

> *What should I do? I have an exclusively breastfed 21 week old baby who I want to do the best for. This is extremely stressful as the evidence is so polarized. I have even received mixed messages from healthcare professionals thus far!*
>
> (Joanne (BBC, 2011))

In 2012 the coalition government introduced yet more assessment of our babies in the UK. The new progress check for all two-year-olds is being carried out under the initiative of offering parents a more detailed update on how their child is progressing. To professionals, the additional assessment for babies at two years of age has been packaged in such a way as to make them believe the check will enable them to spot key indicators of delayed development, delayed speech and other areas of additional need that the child may be presenting. The check will be carried out by health visitors and other professionals working directly with two-year-olds in settings such as preschools and Nurseries.

Critical questions

» *Do parents know that this developmental check for two-year-olds has been introduced?*

» *Do parents understand what the check is aiming to do, or what it is looking for?*

It is doubtful that the majority of parents have any idea what this new intervention is, what it is for or who will carry it out. As a parent myself, no one has talked to me about this assessment and I have two children eligible. Along with the increasing number of immunisations, more and more developmental 'checks' are likely to appear. Our six-year-olds will now be sitting reading tests to ascertain whether they can decode words and non-words, essentially another developmental check. Every check, test and assessment falls in line with the coalition's master plan to improve national averages in schools, improve educational attainment at GCSE and ultimately use our youngest children miraculously to rectify the economic and social ills of the nation.

CASE STUDY

A letter dropped through my door from the team of health visitors whom I hadn't seen since my third child was born, just under five years ago. I've had another child since then. The letter was telling me that they were coming to my home and would be carrying out a progress check on my youngest child. She would have been two-and-a-half at the time. I rang the team and asked if the progress check was the new two-and-a-half-year-old assessment that the government had brought in that year. The health visitor responded that it was indeed that check but that it wasn't new. I was a little shocked because I was aware this progress check was new. Why did she lie to me? I wondered if they had struggled to get parents to undertake the check and so they wanted to make me believe it had always been in place. That was madness in itself because I'd had three children previously and this two-and-a-half-year-old check had never been mentioned before now. It was clearly a lie.

I told the health visitor that we were not having our little girl assessed at two years and that if I thought there were any problems I would raise them with my GP. The response of the health visitor shocks me even now; she said that we would be taken off all future developmental checks. I was astounded. I mean, we didn't want this progress check, but to take us off all future checks – is that how they miss families where children are in need?

I drove home thinking about it. If any parent can call their health visitor and tell them not to come round, and then the health visitor takes the family off the system for further health checks, surely that's how these children on television end up so hurt, or even dead. Like that baby in London, and the one in Birmingham – what if those children's mothers had been taken off all developmental checks?

The system clearly doesn't work, does it?

(Amy, 37)

Power struggles with parents

Another example where parents can be confused as they become entangled in the web created by professionals, all of whom are pursuing what they see as being the very best for children, is in education. Parents will often simply accept what teachers in schools have to say about their child. At parents' evening a teacher may very well state that little Joseph is *near the top end of the profile*, or that quiet Sasha is *right about average, where the government like them to be.* Parents may not have any idea what a 'profile' is or exactly what it means to be 'average'. All parents may wish to know is that their child is behaving at school, following instructions and making something that sounds a lot like progress. Parents see teachers as being the experts.

So if such an important and influential group of people are happy to leave 'schoolification' to the experts, do the experts actually know how much power they yield?

Critical questions

» *Think back to being at school yourself. Was there one particular teacher that you remember as being inspirational? Maybe they first gave you the idea of which career to choose?*

» *Can you think of one teacher where your memories are less favourable, or even negative? Did you ever feel victimised or less favoured by a teacher?*

The job that teachers do every day is not to be mocked; they work long hours, many of which are in their own time. The misconception that teachers have long holidays where time is their own remains a popular myth. Teachers work many week nights in school well past 6pm; they work weekends to support open days, fêtes and charity events; and teachers arrive early and leave late. Holidays are restricted generally to school holiday dates, thus feeding the misconception of extended leave, but in reality many 'school holidays' are spent at conferences and teacher training events, and in preparation for new classes. Teachers work hard, which is not in dispute.

That being said, a child's future, their confidence levels and educational attainment can be entirely dictated by the relationships that they have with one or two teachers across their academic career. Are teachers aware of this huge responsibility? It's doubtful in the main. Despite all the work that teachers do, one small comment that the teacher may make and then never recall again could account for a young child's confidence level dropping to such a degree that they may never recover enough to engage fully with education. Equally, one teacher, and their enthusiasm and ability to teach with individuality in mind, can set a child on course to achieve numerous postgraduate awards and even a doctorate. Consider the two examples below, both recalled clearly by *adults*, both having had a significant impact on the child's academic progress:

Example 1

Year 1 class teacher: I need someone to cut out some shapes.
[Child A raises a hand]
Teacher: Not you, A, I've seen your cutting out ...
[Child A lowers their hand]

Adult reflection

I put my hand down and remember thinking, how does she know what my cutting out is like? I haven't done any in this class yet. She picked Fiona instead of me. Fiona was quiet and shy; everyone liked Fiona. All the teachers liked her. I thought my teacher liked me too, until that day. I never offered to do anything for a teacher after that. Not even once. I was six years old, and that teacher had no idea how much she had hurt my feelings.

Example 2

Year 1 class teacher: Where have you seen purple people?

Adult reflection

I thought I'd done so well drawing the picture. The teacher walked up behind me and told me I had to do it over again. Apparently purple people don't exist and so I shouldn't have coloured them in purple. Even now when my children are drawing it's hard for me to let them colour trees in orange or paint the sky green. All the way back then and I still have an issue with colouring things in exactly how they should be – you know, the real colours ...

The experiences that children have during their early years inside and outside school have a profound and long-term impact on them as adults. Relatively small events in the eyes of a teacher can be enormous in the eyes of a child, and those memories can last a lifetime.

I would argue that parents attending parents' evenings for their own children still walk into school with a little trepidation; they sit quietly listening to the class teacher tell them all about little Sasha or lively Johnny, then they scurry out of the front door hoping the head teacher doesn't catch them. Teachers and head teachers make parents nervous in much the same way they did when those parents were children themselves. The power relationship remains into adulthood, and teachers do little to appreciate the experiences parents may have had in an educational setting, or how they might bridge the ever widening gap between parents and schools.

Critical questions

» *As a teacher, in a school or other setting, how do you expect parents to feel when they walk into your classroom?*

» *Consider how you might reflect upon your own past experiences, and the parents who come to see you. How could you improve your relationship with parents, and in turn with their children?*

Critical reflections

If you ask a parent how they ensure the well-being of their child, they are likely to answer something like:

I think back to when I was a child, I remember some of the things that I did as a child and I know that they shouldn't be doing those things. My fears impact the things that I allow or restrict. For example, I'm not a parent who will let my children run away when we are walking along the side of the road; I have a fear of heights and so I am careful about them being up high. I don't take risks with them; I think my parents took more risks, unnecessary risks. I don't want them to be sheltered to the point that they can't do anything themselves, but I have been more strict about how far they can go out on bikes and how long they are playing out at the weekend. School nights are for homework and time with us as parents so they don't have many extra-curricular activities and that sort of thing. I know that other parents are different; I see them when we go to school. It's not that I think they're wrong and I'm right, but I think I could have done much better as an adult if my parents had taken a little more time with me as a child.

(Alec, 31)

I want them to be happy, healthy and doing well. I want to see them smiling when they see me and enjoying time with us when they're not at school. I hope they enjoy school but it's a necessary evil. I just want them to look back and say they were happy growing up.

(Caroline, 35)

Parents want the best for their children; in 2013 that often means working. In order to work, parents will need their young children to be cared for by an adult other than themselves: grandparents, childminders, Nurseries, nannies etc. How parents choose that person is different for everyone; for every parent the factors surrounding that choice are determined by their own experiences, those around them whom they trust, and the information they are given by government and professionals.

As a professional yourself, what is your contribution to that decision?

Further reading

Greenberg, J.P. (2011) The Impact of Maternal Education on Children's Enrollment in Early Childhood Education and Care. *Children and Youth Services Review*, 33(7): 1049–57.

Greenberg scrutinises just how much the educational experiences and attainment of children's mothers influence families' choice to register their children in some form of early education and care. Using data taken from the National Household Education Survey for a 14-year period the author posits that children are likely to be placed in some sort of childcare if their mother has valued her own educational experiences, and thus a combination of educational advantage and economic advantage enables young children to be registered with higher-quality early-childhood settings, affording them a head start over other children even before beginning formal schooling.

Milteer, R.M.; Ginsberg, K.R.; Mulligan, D.A. (2011) *The Importance of Play in Promoting Healthy Child Development and Maintaining Strong Parent–Child Bond: Focus on Children in Poverty.*

Available from www.ecementor.org/articles-on-teaching/The_Importance_of_Play_in_Promoting_%20Healthy_Child_Development.pdf. Accessed 20 July 2013.

Milteer et al. explore play and child development together as critical elements that are crucial to a child's happy and healthy well-being. The authors hold poverty up as a central reason for the negation of play and development; where young children do not have access to high-quality play experiences, their overall development is impeded. Milteer et al. suggest that there are more than 15 million children under the age of 18 living in the USA who exist in a state of poverty. The authors contend that parents and carers must intervene to ensure that healthy, appropriate play experiences are part of these children's lives, and thus that play mediates the impact of poverty.

Tang, S.; Coley, R.; Votruba-Drzal, E. (2012) Low-Income Families' Selection of Childcare for Their Young Children. *Children and Youth Services Review*, 34: 2002–11.

This journal article reconnoitres the less well-researched area of low-income preschool children attending early childcare in the US. They discuss their results, including the comparison of white mothers and Latino mothers, which suggest that mothers who are in employment, be it full- or part-time, are more likely than mothers who do not work to use non-maternal childcare. This may not in itself be surprising: here in the UK it is often the working mother who engages with external childcare. However, this article considers those who engage with Head Start. These results, when compared to those of our own version, Sure Start, have striking similarities, thus forcing us in the UK to wonder why Sure Start made similar mistakes to Head Start, rather than learning from the US.

3 A health professional's perspective: children's nursing

JACKIE MUSGRAVE

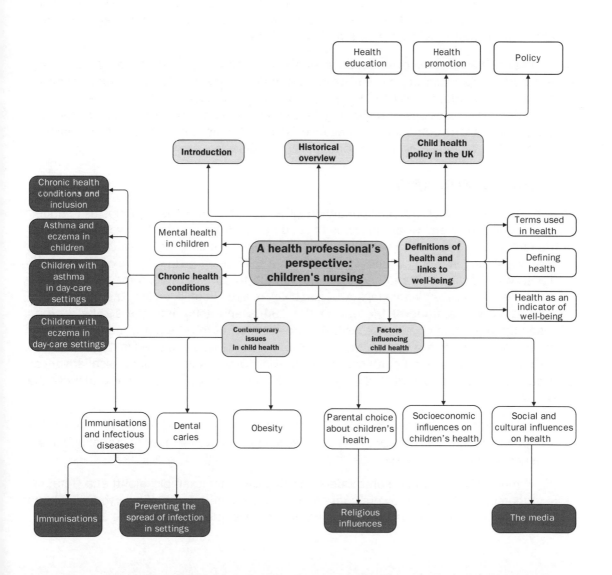

Introduction

This chapter draws on the author's experience as a nurse, in particular of sick children, in order to examine how physical health conditions can impact on children's well-being. In particular, it discusses the contemporary chronic health conditions that affect children in the developed world. It draws on experience gained as a teacher of childcare qualifications in further and higher education, and many of the ideas that are outlined in this chapter reflect discussions with students. It examines the challenges to inclusion that chronic health conditions can bring to professionals who are working with the 2012 Early Years Foundation Stage (EYFS), or indeed any early-childhood education framework. This is an important (and under-researched) area of children's health.

Laevers and Heylen (2003) assess children's levels of emotional well-being as the degree to which children feel at ease, how spontaneously they act, how self-confident they are and how much vitality they exhibit. They also consider children's levels of involvement in activities as an indicator of their emotional well-being. This chapter aims to examine critically how health conditions can challenge children's ability to sustain levels of involvement in activities, and in turn how this may impact on their emotional well-being.

Statham and Chase in their overview of childhood well-being state that *wellbeing is generally understood as the quality of people's lives ... it is understood ... in relation to objective measures, such as ... health status* (2010, p 2). They go on to say that childhood well-being should include physical dimensions of well-being. This statement can be interpreted as suggesting that a physical health condition is a negative factor and may impact on a child's quality of life, and that as a result they may experience a reduced sense of well-being.

Historical overview

To give a broader view of what child health involves, a look back in history helps us to understand why we are where we are in terms of child health. It is important for you to be aware of the factors that can have a positive or negative impact on children's health and, in turn, on their well-being. It is not so long ago that when a child became unwell, the only treatment available was cod liver oil and bed rest. The limited treatment options meant that many children died or were left with a legacy of disability as a result of illnesses. The post-Second World War period, starting at the end of the 1940s and going into the 1950s, saw an intense period of medical advancement that meant that there were many more options for treatment available. In the UK, the National Health Service was launched in 1948, and this offered, and still does, free health-care to all citizens. Other examples of medical advances that have contributed to reducing child mortality and improving child health include the following.

*   *Antibiotics* were discovered in the 1940s, and this meant that the death rate among young children was reduced because treatment was available for bacterial infections such as pneumonia and meningitis.

*   *Immunisations* against some infectious diseases (for example diphtheria, tetanus, tuberculosis, polio) that were common causes of death or disability in young children (and still are dangerous to young children) first became available in the 1950s.

- *Paediatric surgery* became safer in this period. This was partly because surgeons started to take an interest in children's surgery and it became a specialist branch of medicine. Part of the reason for the increased safety and improved success of paediatric surgery was improved and safer anaesthetics developed for children. The expertise that was developed meant that life-saving or life-enhancing surgery could be carried out for the first time. Thus children with congenital heart defects (meaning that the defect was present at birth) could receive an operation to correct the problem, which previously would have resulted in death or a life of disability.

- *Neonatal medicine*, the care of new-born babies, became a specialism in the 1950s when the first special care baby unit was opened in Bristol. Before this time there was limited treatment available for babies who had difficult births, or were born early or with congenital conditions. Neonatal medicine dramatically improved the survival rate of sick babies at this vulnerable stage.

These medical milestones meant there was a significant reduction in the death rate among young children. As the last century progressed, there were advances in the understanding of the causes of diseases and the effects on health (epidemiology), and this meant a shift away from disease cure to disease prevention.

Critical question

» *Consider the challenges that the health profession has faced over the past 60 years and identify some of the conditions where treatment is now available. Critically compare the health profession and access to health-care at points over the past 100 years.*

Child health policy in the UK

Preventing disease and ill health is approached by health education and health promotion interventions, and both of these concepts are key to the provision of child health policy in the UK; therefore it is important to have an understanding of what the terms mean.

Health education

This involves methods used to teach people about the causes of illness and poor health. The importance of health education is reflected in the UK school education system. In the early years, EYFS professionals are expected to ensure that children *know the importance of good health* (DfE, 2012, p 8). Children aged five upwards receive health education as part of the school curriculum through personal, social and health education (PSHE).

Health promotion

This is defined by Hall and Elliman (2006, p 6) as *any planned and informed intervention which is designed to improve physical or mental health or prevent disease, disability or premature death*. Examples of health promotion activities for children include immunisations and the two-year-old check.

Policy

The last decade has seen a policy focus on the health of children in the UK. Below is a list of the main policies, in date order. You should familiarise yourself with these.

*   The *Every Child Matters Agenda* (2003) advocates a multiagency approach in order to provide all services for children.

*   The National Service Framework for Children (DH, 2004) was developed in response to the Every Child Matters agenda, and is a ten-year programme designed to improve the health and well-being of children and young people. The framework set the standards for all service providers.

*   *Managing Medicines in Schools and Early Years Settings* is guidance for all professionals and families to work together to ensure that *children requiring medicines receive the support they need* (DH and DfES, 2005, p 1).

*   The Healthy Child Programme (DH, 2009) is a significant policy that plays a key role in *improving the health and well being of children* (p 5). The Programme offers *universal* and *targeted* services for children, aimed at health promotion and prevention. Policy priorities focus on reducing obesity in the early years, improving dental health and promoting the uptake of immunisations.

*   *Supporting Families in the Foundation Years* (DfE and DH, 2011) states that *children's health is strongly influenced by what happens in the womb and the first two years of life* (p 9). The policy outlines how parents and professionals, especially Early Years Professionals (EYPs) and health visitors, can work together to improve health outcomes.

*   The revised EYFS (DfE, 2012b) demonstrates how recent policy is striving to achieve a joined-up thinking approach between the Healthy Child Programme and the EYFS by offering a universal service to children with a developmental and health check for two-year-olds in order to achieve the aims of the Every Child Matters agenda. The two-year-old check is an example of a *universal* service using a multiagency approach. EYPs conduct two-year-old development checks aimed at promoting the outcomes of the EYFS by checking that the development of each child is as expected. The developmental two-year-old check assessment informs the health check and is conducted by health visitors in order to meet the aims of the Healthy Child Programme. The findings from the two-year-old check may result in children being referred for *targeted* services in order to put interventions in place aimed at promoting development. At the time of writing, there is an integrated review being conducted in order to identify the most effective approach to conducting the two-year-old check.

*   *Social and Emotional Well-being: Early Years* (NICE, 2012) is the National Institute for Health and Clinical Excellence's (NICE) endorsement of the value of early interventions in order to promote the well-being of children in the early years. The role of professionals who care for and educate babies and young children is critical to the government policy to promote well-being.

*   *Conception to Age 2: The Age of Opportunity* (Wave Trust and DfE, 2013) is an addendum to the government's vision for the foundation years, *Supporting Families*

in the Foundation Years (DfE and DH, 2011). The report is the product of a Special Interest Group for children from conception to age two, and aims to improve child development outcomes through better support from professionals for the families who need the most support.

Definitions of health and links to well-being

Terms used in health

There are increasing numbers of children with health needs in early years settings and, as a practitioner, you will play a vital role in maintaining and promoting the health of children. Many professionals are extending their knowledge and skills in order to be able to identify and meet the health needs of children, and so create an inclusive environment. An understanding of common terms will be helpful to you; below are some broad descriptions of health conditions.

•   *Acute* describes a health condition of rapid onset. It can be severe, for instance an infection such as meningitis, or a less severe condition caused by a virus, like the common cold.

•   *Chronic* describes a disease of long duration involving very slow changes.

•   *Complex medical needs*, as the term suggests, include a range of conditions that may be the result of a child being born prematurely. This can mean that the organs of the body have not developed as expected. Interventions (such as medicine or physiotherapy) may be required to maintain as healthy a life as possible, or sometimes to maintain life.

Defining health

Professionals frequently talk about children's health, but this is often in the context of 'being healthy' or 'healthy eating'. The revised EYFS states that *children learn best when they are healthy* (DfE, 2012, p 13). But what does being healthy mean? The most commonly used definition of health comes from the World Health Organization (WHO):

> *The extent to which an individual or group is able on the one hand to realise the aspirations and satisfy needs; and, on the other hand,* to change or cope with the environment. *Health is, therefore, seen as a resource for everyday life, not the objective of living; it is a positive concept emphasising social and personal resources, as well as physical capacities.*

(WHO, 1986)

The words *to change or cope with the environment* have been emphasised because they are significant to EYPs. This is because many health conditions do not have a cure, and the children require intervention, such as inhalers or other medication, in order to remove or minimise the symptoms of the condition. Alternatively, the child's environment may need to be changed in order to help them cope. An example of this could be if a child has anaphylaxis (a severe allergy) to a common food product such as lactose (in milk). Then you would need to consider how to make the environment free from lactose in order to prevent the child from coming into contact with the allergy-causing substance. This in turn reduces the symptoms of the condition that can cause the child to feel ill or to experience poor health. If children are helped in this way to achieve the best level of health, they can experience good levels of well-being, thus increasing their disposition to participate in activities and to learn. This point is returned to in the section below that discusses asthma and the implications for practice.

Critical question

» *Critically evaluate the definition from your position. How does it reflect your role in promoting or maintaining the health of the children you are caring for and educating?*

Health as an indicator of well-being

Well-being is defined in the *Oxford English Dictionary* as *the state of being comfortable, healthy or happy*. This is a simplistic definition; however, it does illustrate that children need to experience good health in order to develop good well-being, and hopefully this will help them to be happier.

If you consider Laevers and Heylen's (2003) view that children's levels of well-being are reflected in their level of involvement in activities, it is easy to see that the presence of symptoms caused by a health condition may result in a lack of involvement. For example, tiredness can interfere with concentration levels; in turn this can cause a lack of vitality and, consequently, a lack of involvement. From your own perspective, perhaps you can reflect on a time when you have had a common cold virus. The usual symptoms include sore throat, raised body temperature, headache, sneezing, runny nose, lack of appetite, lethargy and tiredness. As an adult, you are in a position to respond by taking regular medication such as paracetamol, which can be used effectively to reduce many of these symptoms.

Now consider the effect of a common cold from the perspective of young children. How are they likely to feel if they are starting a cold? Probably not that much different from the way that you feel, but how do they convey their feelings of being unwell? How may a viral illness affect their behaviour? Having a cold will probably affect their involvement in activities as well as their disposition for learning and general vitality. However, the symptoms and impact on children's daily living caused by a cold virus will usually be short-lived, and after a few days they will recover their normal level of health and return to feeling well enough to engage with their usual activities. This may not be the situation for children with a chronic health condition because the symptoms can be ongoing, and as a consequence can have a long-term impact on daily life.

Factors influencing child health

As a practitioner, you should view children's learning in the context of social and cultural factors. It is also important to consider these factors in relation to health-related issues. This will involve you getting to know children and their families in order to gain an understanding of their health beliefs and an insight into why some parents may not appear to be doing the best they can for their children's health.

This section aims to highlight just a few of the many influences on children's health, which can include:

* parental decisions and choices;

* socioeconomic effects;

* sociocultural influences;

* family lifestyles;

* media;

* religious influences.

Parental choice about children's health

It can be difficult to reconcile yourself with parental choices about children's health when it is clear to you that these choices are having a negative impact, sometimes to the extent that children do not enjoy optimal levels of health. In extreme cases, parental choice may result in disability or death. In these cases, children who are denied medical treatment because of parental choice will become cases for safeguarding processes.

Denying a child optimal health contradicts everything that one aims and hopes for when working with and caring for sick children. As a practitioner you will want the best for the children for whom you are professionally responsible, and it can be hard to accept the fact that some parents do not actively take up services aimed at improving their child's health.

Parents can deny their child a right to health in the following ways:

* *actively* refusing medical help: for example a parent who refuses to administer medication because of religious beliefs;

* *inactively* denying a child optimal health: for example when parents do not take up the offer of universal services because of inertia. This may be as a result of lifestyle choices associated with substance misuse, which renders parents unable to summon the energy to take their child for a service such as immunisation.

The reasons that parents may make such a choice are complex and probably very difficult to overcome. It is vital that you continue to work with parents and preserve a relationship that remains focused on the well-being of their child.

Equally, it is essential that your personal views are not voiced and that judgements about parents' actions are suspended.

Socioeconomic influences on children's health

We live in a world where many children live in poverty and, as Underdown (2007, p 57) asserts, *poverty is the greatest threat to children's health worldwide*. Underdown goes on to make a distinction between living in poverty in a poor country and living in poverty in a rich country. There are stark differences in children's health between the poor and rich nations of the world. People who live in absolute poverty in the poor countries of the world frequently do not have access to health-care, nor is there the infrastructure to provide clean water and sanitation. An absence of these resources and the lack of adequate nutrition because of famine conditions have a negative effect on children's health. In addition to these factors, the presence of malaria is a constant threat.

Solutions to try and improve health by reducing poverty are the focus of the United Nations (UN) Millennium Development Goals (MDGs). The UN Report (2011) suggests that the MDGs are having a positive effect on reducing poverty. One way that this is being achieved is by offering immunisations and establishing controls to reduce the spread of infectious diseases. These measures help to optimise health for children and reduce the level of disability, which can be a legacy of disease. In turn this increases well-being, as well as helping to develop adults who are more able to work and make a contribution to society – a further contributory factor to increased well-being.

Despite the current economic climate, the UK is still one of the richest countries in the world. However, there are many families living in relative poverty, which is defined as children living in households earning less than 60 per cent of the national median income. In some areas of England as many as 47 per cent of children can be living in poverty. This can have a detrimental effect on children's health, because providing a balanced and healthy diet is often neglected when money is short. Eating unhealthy food predisposes children to becoming obese and developing dental decay (caries).

Even in relatively well-off families, children's health can be affected negatively if parents work long hours, meaning that they find it difficult to access health services. As a consequence, their children may miss out on these. Families who are 'cash rich' but 'time poor' may buy expensive convenience foods, and therefore the children miss out on fresh and nutritious food.

However, it is not just availability of money that influences children's health, and the following sections explore other relevant factors.

Social and cultural influences on health

One group in society who experience poorer health outcomes are Gypsy, Roma and Travelling (GRT) communities. Wilkin et al. (2009) conducted a literature review in order to highlight some of the difficulties faced by GRT children. The purpose of the review was to identify ways of improving their educational outcomes; however, the review highlights that GRT people not only have low educational outcomes – they also have poorer health. This is partly because of a reluctance to engage with health services. The reasons for such reluctance are not difficult to understand if you examine the social and cultural context of their lives. By definition, many GRT families move around from place to place, and this can make it difficult to access health services. It can also result in difficulties associated with keeping records of the health services that have been delivered, thus increasing the chances of important health-care services, such as immunisations, not being available to these children or not being recorded accurately.

In addition to the practical difficulty of accessing and having records of child health, GRT families have suffered from prejudice and the effects of negative stereotypes throughout history, and it is suggested that this has resulted in a wariness of professionals. There is also a reluctance to discuss health issues with strangers. These factors all contribute to GRT communities' experiencing health problems that are two to five times more common than in non-GRT families (Parry et al., 2004).

Immigration is another sociocultural factor that may result in parents being reluctant to accept health services for their children. People who have lived in countries where organised health services are not available may find the highly structured approach offered by the NHS complex and confusing. In order to gain insight into this point, imagine that you have moved from a war-torn country in a developing part of the world, where there are few health services and where doctors are only consulted when somebody is unwell. In addition to this, the cost of consulting medical treatment is prohibitive. Imagine that you arrive in the UK, where you are expected to take your healthy baby for check-ups that are centred around early intervention. The reasons why parents may have difficulties in adapting to the complexity of healthcare in the UK are not difficult to appreciate.

The media

The media have major influences on children's health. To illustrate this point, Anderson and Anderson (2010) conducted research into the messages about food that are conveyed to children in preschool television programmes. They selected a range of programmes broadcast on a Canadian television channel aimed at children between the ages of two and five years in order to analyse the references to food and eating in the programme content. They found that there was a prevalence of references to high-fat and high-sugar foods, such as cookies, cake and pie. Some of the storylines portrayed characters going to great lengths to pursue sweets as a prize. Another storyline portrayed a character who was rewarded for hard work with repeated offers of chocolate pudding. Anderson and Anderson assert that such reinforcements communicate the message to children that these foods are desirable. This research suggests that preschool children are vulnerable to messages conveyed to them by television characters. If you think about how food manufacturers use children's characters on packaging in order to promote their foods and make them appealing to children, it suggests that media can influence children's selection of food products in powerful ways. If the products tend to be non-nutritious, or they are of low nutritional value, then it follows that the media can have a negative influence on children's health.

Critical questions

»   *What role can you play in minimising the negative impact of media influences on children's diets?*

»   *Critically evaluate how you reinforce positive messages about nutritious foods in your setting. How might this be improved or shared with other professionals?*

Religious influences

The choices that parents make in relation to their children's health can be influenced by religious beliefs. For example, Christian Scientists do not believe in accessing conventional medical services. The leader of the church in 1983 stated that children who were sick would be prayed for, rather than offered medical treatment. Another well-known example is Jehovah's Witnesses' refusal of blood transfusions, even if this results in death. The belief is derived from their interpretation of the Bible's teaching that a human being must not sustain their own life with the blood of another creature (Acts 15:20, 28–29). By accepting another person's blood the recipient risks losing eternal life (Schott and Henley, 1996).

It may be difficult to comprehend such deeply held religious beliefs, and if the beliefs are held by a minority of people it can be more difficult to accept that a parent could risk their child's health. However, faith and religious observance can be a positive factor for individuals' well-being. If a major religious teaching is not adhered to, as in the health-related examples cited here, this may lead to feelings of guilt and resentment – negative emotions that can result in reduced well-being.

Critical questions

» *Consider some of the children and their families that you have had experience of working with.*

» *Appraise your own views of child health.*

» *Imagine a scenario linked to one of the influences discussed above, where you may have a different opinion from a family or parents. How could you prepare yourself to respond to it?*

» *How would you support other professionals in coping with such a situation in your setting?*

Contemporary issues in child health

As outlined above, current UK child health policy is aimed at providing *universal* services for all children. If, as a result of having a universal service – for example the two-year-old check – children and families deemed to be at a disadvantage or vulnerable are then offered further intervention, this is described as a *targeted* service. The targets of policies for improving child health include the following areas:

• obesity;

• dental decay;

• immunisations and infectious diseases;

• mental health.

Obesity

Obesity is described as the most common nutritional disorder of recent years in western societies (Oxford Medical Dictionary, 2010). The extent of the problem is so great that Hall and Elliman (2006, p 179) state that the term *epidemic of obesity* is used with justification. People carrying an excess of weight can find taking part in physical exercise more difficult and less pleasurable (imagine how you would feel if you were asked to carry a 2kg bag of potatoes with you for a day); therefore less physical activity and an intake of surplus calories creates a vicious circle that is difficult to break.

There are short- and long-term considerations about the links between obesity and well-being. In the short term, during the early years, there are issues relating to inclusion to be considered. For example, children who are obese can be reluctant to engage in physical activity because they find running around causes them discomfort from shortness of breath or tiredness. This can mean that they are excluded from play activities because they do not have the same level of physical stamina. However, it is not just physical outdoor activities that can be difficult. A Foundation Degree student chose childhood obesity as the subject of an assignment because she noticed that a three-year-old in her setting had difficulty sitting down on the floor and crossing her legs. This meant that she had to sit on a chair away from the other children. Even an everyday activity, then, such as sitting on the floor with other children, becomes an uncomfortable experience and can result in being treated differently.

There are probably many more examples of how obesity can impact on children in the early years, and you will have many that you can think of. The consequences of being treated differently as a result of obesity require further consideration. For example, if children find outdoor play too strenuous this can result in exclusion from social play experiences. As well as social exclusion, if children are unable to take part in physical activities that are planned as part of the curriculum, they are also being excluded from their education. The effects of exclusion can lead to feelings of isolation and reduced levels of social and emotional development. As previously stated, poor social and emotional development causes individuals to experience lower levels of well-being.

There are also long-term considerations about the impact of obesity in the early years because obese children are very likely to become obese adults. As well as the health concerns that are related to obesity (high blood pressure, diabetes and heart disease, to name a few), there are associated emotional and social implications, as well as increased levels of depression and obesity.

Critical questions

» *Childhood obesity is a sensitive subject, and as a professional it is essential that you handle interventions in settings ethically: that is, without causing harm by attempting to address children's eating habits with parents.*

» *How could you employ appropriate interventions aimed at promoting children's healthy eating and increased physical activity?*

» *How can you work in partnership with parents in an ethical way?*

Dental caries

Dental caries, or decay, is when the enamel of the teeth is broken down, and the most common cause is the acid formed by the bacterial breakdown of sugar in the diet. If dental decay is not prevented, or there is no treatment, teeth continue to be damaged, and a tooth abscess and extreme pain can be the outcome. This is obviously an unnecessary source of suffering for children. However, the incidence of dental decay is increasing, with 40 per cent of five-year-olds shown to have active tooth decay. Children are entitled to free dental care in England; however, only 60 per cent of three-to-five-year-olds are registered with a dentist.

Eating and drinking foods containing sugar cause the increased incidence of dental decay, and some of this increase may be linked to the consumption of sugary drinks. Such is the extent of the problem that, at the time of writing, the government is considering taxation on sugary drinks in order to deter consumers from purchasing them.

Critical questions

» *How can you promote good dental hygiene in your setting?*

» *How do you think good dental hygiene links to well-being?*

Immunisations and infectious diseases

Infections are caused by the spread of bacteria, viruses and fungi. Infectious diseases can be fatal at worst, or a significant inconvenience if an acute infection, such as norovirus, is contracted. Many infectious diseases can be avoided, or at least minimised, in the following ways:

• administering immunisations against a range of infectious diseases, such as polio, diphtheria, tetanus, whooping cough, measles, mumps and rubella;

• implementing measures aimed at preventing the spread of infection.

Up-to-date information about immunisations and the control of infection can be obtained from the Public Health England (PHE) website (PHE, 2013a).

Immunisations

Immunisations are life-saving and can reduce the risk of disabilities in children resulting from contraction of an infectious disease, but there are many reasons why parents may not take up the immunisation services. Consider immunisations in the context of the section above that explored the influences on parents' choices about their children's health.

Many infectious diseases that once commonly caused death and disability are now largely avoidable in the UK because of free immunisations. The Health Protection Agency (HPA; part of PHE since April 2013) has up-to-date information about the current immunisation (or vaccination) schedule that is available (PHE, 2013b). Polio (and many other infectious diseases) can leave a legacy of disability and pain, both of which are factors linked to poor well-being. However, immunisation uptake has not been as good as it could be in recent years, and government immunisation targets have not been achieved. One reason for the lower levels of uptake is the recent controversy about the safety of immunisations; in particular, the measles, mumps and rubella (MMR) vaccine was widely reported as a suspected cause of autism. Even though the research that caused people to lose confidence in immunisations has been discredited, and the doctor responsible has been struck off the medical register because of his actions, some people remain suspicious about the safety of immunisations. The incidence of measles has increased, and this is partly because parents are not taking up the offer of immunisation for their children. Measles can lead to chronic ear infections, and in turn these can lead to speech- and language-development delay. In rare cases, measles can lead to brain damage and can be fatal.

Most children can receive immunisations safely, and it is vital that parents understand the possible implications of not having their children immunised.

Critical questions

»   *What is your role in educating parents about the importance of immunisations for their children?*

»   *Consider the ethics of immunisations. Do you think that you have a responsibility to protect all children in your setting by promoting immunisations?*

»   *In the United States, children have to be immunised before they are allowed to start school. Do you think that this is an approach that could be adopted in the UK to ensure that parents have their children immunised? How might this impede parental choice?*

»   *How do you balance parental choice in relation to immunisations? How do you suspend personal views?*

Preventing the spread of infection in settings

There are two main ways to prevent the spread of infection in day-care settings.

•   Individuals need to adopt high standards of personal hygiene, especially the use of good hand-washing techniques.

•   It is important to maintain a clean environment.

There are many infectious diseases for which there is no available immunisation via the NHS immunisation schedule: for example hand, foot and mouth disease, and the common cold. The effects of infectious diseases can have a profound impact on well-being, as discussed above. Less visible is the effect on both children's and adults' well-being created by higher incidence of sick leave, which can cause increased workload for adults, as well as staff changes, resulting in unrest for children. Therefore there are compelling reasons for ensuring that the spread of infection in settings is minimised.

The primary means by which the organisms that cause infections are spread is hand contact. Therefore the most effective way of reducing the spread of infection is to remove organisms from hands using effective hand-washing techniques. It is important to bear in mind that the use of disposable gloves does not remove the need for effective hand-washing. In fact, the use of gloves can give a false sense of security and it is important that gloves are used with care. Children need to be taught about these important aspects of minimising the spread of infection from a very early age. A valuable way to teach children good hand-washing habits is through professionals modelling good practice and incorporating effective hand-washing into the routines of the setting.

There have been many media reports about the increase in meticillin-resistant *Staphylococcus aureus* (MRSA) infections. Understandably, such reports can cause alarm. However, *Staphylococcus* is a common type of bacterium and is often present on the skin, and in the nose and throat; it can cause impetigo. In extreme cases, if it enters the bloodstream through a cut, it can cause blood-poisoning and requires a course of antibiotics.

However, some strains of *Staphylococcus* have become resistant to antibiotics, resulting in cases of MRSA. Reasons that *Staphylococcus* has become resistant to antibiotics include:

•   the overuse of antibiotics for infections that would have improved without them;

•   prescribed courses of antibiotics not being completed;

•   the ability of strains of bacteria to mutate and become resistant to antibiotics over time.

This is a serious problem, and recent reports have suggested that drug companies are not investing money in developing new antibiotics because there is less profit to be made than in other areas of research.

Despite this alarming situation, it may be surprising that healthy individuals are at low risk of becoming infected with MRSA. Public Health England does not advise the exclusion of individuals with MRSA from day-care settings. Key to preventing the spread of MRSA is the maintenance of a hygienic environment and adherence to effective hand-washing routines. However, some children are more vulnerable than others to contracting MRSA.

CASE STUDY

Ethan's story

Ethan is three, and he was born with a condition that means he has complex medical needs. Ethan has been into hospital for several operations to correct some of the problems he has as a result of the condition. His most recent operation was to repair his palate so that hopefully he can eat normal food in the future rather than being fed via his gastric feeding tube. During the hospital stay, Ethan's parents were informed that he had MRSA. He made a rapid recovery from his operation and wanted to return to nursery. The medical staff explained to Ethan's parents that there was little risk of the MRSA affecting other children and staff at the nursery. However, the staff were very unhappy about Ethan returning because of their concerns about MRSA.

Critical questions

Imagine you are the manager of the nursery and consider the following.

»   *How are you going to explain the facts to staff?*

»   *How are you going to reassure them?*

»   *How might you deal with the situation in relation to other parents?*

»   *How are you going to ensure that all staff work to policies that are aimed at maintaining good standards of hygiene and practice?*

Bear in mind that it is possible a child could have an infectious disease such as MRSA or HIV, but this fact may not have been disclosed to you. Therefore, it is essential that good standards of personal and environmental hygiene be maintained, especially when you come into contact with bodily fluids, in order to protect all individuals.

Mental health in children

The WHO defines mental health as *a state of well-being in which the individual realises his or her own abilities, can cope with the normal stresses of life, can work productively and fruitfully, and is able to make a contribution to his or her community* (WHO, 2007).

Promoting good mental health is beneficial to individuals and to society. Poor mental health reduces individuals' ability to cope with life. Anxiety and depression are two common symptoms of poor mental health, and it is not difficult to appreciate how experiencing these symptoms can be a barrier to being 'productive and fruitful'. Reduced productivity as a result of mental health means that individuals may be unable to work, thus reducing the contribution they can make to society. In addition to this, poor mental health may require individuals to access health services and medication, which is an additional financial cost.

In recent years, mental health issues in children have become a cause for concern in the developed world. Some of the reasons for deteriorating levels of mental health are thought to be the effects of competitive education, family breakdown and commercial marketing on children. Department of Health (DH) figures suggest that as many as one in ten children and young people have *some kind of diagnosable mental disorder* that is severe enough to require referral to specialist services (DH, 2007, p 52). An example of a diagnosable condition is depression, which is estimated to affect as many as 10 per cent of five-to-16-year-old children. The increasing numbers have caused de Braal (2009) to question if there is an epidemic of depression. The fact that 10 per cent of children and young people require professional intervention is worrying; however, what is not known is the number of children and young people who are not diagnosed with mental health conditions and yet still experience symptoms such as anxiety and depression.

The trend of increasing numbers of children with mental health issues has prompted policies to attempt to stem the problem. The Healthy Child Programme (2009) aims to provide universal services in order to offer early intervention and put preventative measures in place. There is an abundance of evidence indicating that babies need to be able to develop good-quality relationships and secure attachments in order to have good social and emotional development, which in turn helps individuals to have good mental health. The focus on the importance of enabling babies to develop good emotional and social well-being in order to promote good mental health is a theme in government child health policies over the last ten years.

Critical questions

» *Drawing upon current interpretations of developmental theories, how does your practice address the need to promote children's social and emotional development?*

» *How can you work sensitively with parents to try and achieve this aim?*

Chronic health conditions

This section examines common chronic health conditions that can affect children in the developed world.

Brown et al. (1995) define chronic conditions as those that last for more than three months and are incurable; the effects can have a significant impact on the lives of children and can

Table 3 *A summary of chronic health conditions in the developed world*

Condition	Definition	Symptoms
Anaphylaxis (severe allergy)	An emergency condition resulting from an abnormal and immediate allergic response to a substance to which the body has become allergic.	Flushing; itching; nausea and vomiting; swelling of the mouth, tongue and airway enough to cause an obstruction; wheezing; low blood pressure. On occasions can be fatal.
Asthma	Narrowing of the airways caused by an inflammatory response to a trigger (a substance that can provoke asthma symptoms). Common triggers include animal hair, dust, chemicals, exercise, viruses, pollen.	Wheeze, cough (especially at night), shortness of breath.
Diabetes mellitus	A condition where the pancreas fails to produce adequate amounts of the hormone insulin, which is required to metabolise carbohydrate.	Not enough insulin can result in the blood sugar level rising (hyperglycaemia), and causes thirst and the production of large amounts of urine. Too much insulin (and/or physical exercise) can result in lowering of the blood sugar level (hypoglycaemia); this is a first aid emergency that requires sugar to be given to increase blood sugar level and avoid coma.
Eczema	A common skin condition that is often associated with asthma and allergy.	Eczema is from the Greek meaning *to boil* and is characterised by blisters and weals on the skin that can burst and then crust over, causing intense and painful itching.
Epilepsy	A disorder of brain function that can result in seizures or fits. There is a wide range of causes, and the impact on the individual is influenced by the cause of the brain dysfunction and the location of the damage or disorder in the brain.	Individuals can experience *major* seizures, where the individual falls to the ground and experiences spasms, often accompanied by blueness of the skin, incontinence and convulsions; or *absence* seizures, most common in children, resulting in unconsciousness for a few seconds, which can be accompanied by twitching of the fingers and fluttering of the eyelids. Children may have learning difficulties.
Sickle cell anaemia	An inherited blood condition that commonly affects children of African ancestry but can affect those of Mediterranean, Indian and Saudi Arabian ancestry. Red blood cells are abnormally formed, and when starved of oxygen they form crystals causing them to become an abnormal 'sickle' (or crescent) shape.	The abnormally shaped 'sickle' cells clump and become distorted, which can block up the small vessels, known as sickling. This can cause swelling and intense pain, leading to a sickle cell crisis.

interfere with normal childhood activity. Children who have a chronic health condition are very likely to have symptoms that require intervention in order to maintain or promote good health, and how well this is achieved is a significant factor in their level of well-being.

Children with chronic health conditions will require medical intervention from their GP or hospital consultant; advice on how to give medication or treatment may be given by specialist nurses. Therefore, it is likely that several health professionals are involved in passing on information to the parents of children with chronic conditions. In turn, relevant information needs to be passed on to those who care for and educate young children in day-care settings. Professionals need to understand how symptoms of chronic health conditions can be provoked (or triggered) and, conversely, they need to know what can be done to adapt the environment for children to minimise the effect of the symptoms. These points will be examined in more detail in sections below.

Further information on how to manage these conditions can be found in the guidance *Managing Medicines in Schools and Early Years Settings* (DfES and DH, 2005), which includes information about anaphylaxis, asthma, diabetes and epilepsy. However, the guidance does not include information about eczema, which is thought to affect 20 per cent of children in the UK. The National Eczema Society has produced an activity pack for schools; the details of how to locate this are given in the reference list. The pack is aimed at encouraging discussion about eczema, and the age range it addresses is from four to 11. This leaves a gap in the information that is available for children from birth to the age of three. Because there are so many children affected by eczema and there is a lack of information available, there is a section below that focuses on some of the issues relating to young children with eczema.

Critical question

»   *How can you work effectively with parents to ensure that the health needs of children with chronic health conditions are incorporated into their routines?*

Chronic health conditions and inclusion

The signs and symptoms of some chronic conditions can mean that not all activities are suitable for the children who have them, and they may therefore be excluded from aspects of the curriculum. This section examines how chronic health symptoms, inclusion and well-being are linked together.

The philosophy of inclusion is embedded in UK education policy, and the revised EYFS states its aim for professionals to provide *equality of opportunity and anti-discriminatory practice, ensuring that every child is included and supported* (DfE, 2012b, p 2). This statement reflects Nutbrown and Clough's view of what inclusion is, which they summarise as *maximal participation, minimal exclusion from early years, schools and society* (Nutbrown and Clough, 2006, p 3). However, there are challenges to inclusive practice for practitioners implementing the EYFS, and if inclusion is not achieved, then a child's sense of well-being can be affected in a negative way.

Many professionals have used their knowledge and wisdom to develop their practice so that activities and the environment are inclusive for children with chronic conditions. This means that these children are included in their curriculum and their early years setting (and in society), and that they have opportunities to reach good levels of development, which can give them a sense of achievement. In turn, this links to a sense of children developing 'good' well-being.

Conversely, being excluded can lead to a sense of 'poor' well-being and, as a consequence, children may not achieve their potential social and emotional developmental outcomes. The NICE guidance for social and emotional well-being in the early years states: *poor social and emotional capabilities increase the likelihood of antisocial behaviour and mental health problems, substance abuse, teenage pregnancy, poor educational attainment and involvement in criminal activity* (NICE, 2012, p 18).

Asthma and eczema in children

Asthma and eczema are the two most common chronic conditions that affect children; 20 per cent of children have eczema and between 10 and 15 per cent have asthma. Therefore, the following sections will focus on gaining an understanding of the implications for inclusion for children with asthma and eczema.

Children with asthma in day-care settings

Asthma is an inflammatory condition of the airways; it is common, affecting many children in the UK, and can cause sufferers to feel very unwell and unhealthy. Asthma in very rare cases is fatal; however, the adults in the lives of children who have asthma can help to minimise its symptoms: wheezing, coughing and shortness of breath. There are two ways that asthma symptoms can be reduced in order to help a child to feel healthier and, in turn, this will help to increase feelings of well-being.

* Asthma symptoms can be provoked, or 'triggered', by substances such as animal hair, house-dust mites, emotional stress and physical exercise. Therefore, adapting the environment in order to remove or reduce the presence of triggers is an example of how *the environment can be changed* in order to promote the health of children with asthma.

* Medication with regular inhalers can help to relieve the inflammation and therefore open up the airways, thus reducing the classic symptoms of asthma; this in turn helps children to *cope with the environment*.

Critical question

» *How can you adapt the environment of your setting for children with asthma in order to help them cope?*

Children with eczema in day-care settings

Eczema is an inflammatory condition and it often runs in families. It is associated with allergy, and it is common for children who have eczema also to have asthma and allergy (or anaphylaxis) to food or substances such as animal hair or latex. Eczema is the most common reason why children under the age of two are taken to see their general practitioner in the developed world.

The word *eczema* comes from the Greek word meaning *to boil*. Any of you who have had experience of this skin condition will appreciate that the skin can feel as if it is boiling when it comes into contact with substances that cause a reaction. Such a reaction causes red weals to form on the skin; the weals quickly burst and the skin becomes intensely itchy. People with eczema will find momentary relief in scratching; children may scratch with such intensity that they cause themselves to bleed. When skin is broken in this way, infection can easily enter the body and antibiotics are required in order to treat infection. Eczema is a condition that can have a serious impact on a child's health, and as a consequence it can be a negative influence on well-being. In order to gain an insight into the effects on a small baby of having eczema, read the following case study and reflect on the questions posed.

CASE STUDY

Josh's story

Josh is eight months old and he has attended his day-care setting for five months. He was diagnosed with eczema when he was four months old. Josh has angry-looking areas of eczema on his face. He also has large patches on his knees, ankles, hands, wrists and elbows. He is sitting in a baby seat and is watching the busy setting with deep interest. From time to time he rubs his cheeks against the side of the baby seat, which makes his cheeks look redder and more inflamed. On his hands he is wearing cotton mittens to stop him from scratching the patches of eczema with his finger nails. However, he rubs his hands against his skin frequently and only stops when he is distracted by something that claims his attention. Josh's key person, Becky, says that when he is picked up for a cuddle he will rub parts of his body vigorously against her in order to relieve the itchiness.

The cotton mittens are removed when Becky can sit with him and play. This is usually during meal and snack times when she hands over the supervision of feeding the other children in her key group to colleagues so that she can spend time one to one with Josh. Becky knows that Josh will take any opportunity to scratch, and if allowed to do so will make himself bleed. Becky has worked with Josh's mum and together they have devised this approach to caring for Josh in order to prevent him from damaging his skin and to avoid the possibility of his developing an infection. There is also a health-and-safety consideration to bear in mind: if Josh makes himself bleed as a result of scratching himself, this is a potential risk to people in the setting. And there is a careful balance to be maintained between keeping Josh healthy and comfortable and promoting his development. Becky is concerned about Josh's fine motor development, and she has carried out observations of Josh to assess the level he has reached. She is aware that Josh, at the age of nine months, needs opportunities to develop his pincer grip; however, the presence of the cotton mittens means that he may be denied some essential opportunities to do so.

Critical questions

» *Comment on the effect of Josh's health on his well-being by considering both Josh's and Becky's perspectives.*

From Josh's perspective

Imagine that you are eight months old, your arms are too short to reach the furthest part of your body such as your ankles, they are really itchy and you want to scratch them. How do you think you would feel and what do you think would make you feel better?

From Becky's perspective

Josh's parents and Becky have worked together and taken advice from medical staff to create an approach that is aimed at keeping him as well as possible. However, how do you balance this approach to keeping his skin healthy with minimising the potential negative impact on his development? At nine months, babies should be developing their fine motor skills, especially their pincer grip.

» *How can you plan appropriate activities for Josh?*

» *How can you identify Josh's needs so that you keep him comfortable and prevent him from scratching?*

» *How can you plan for his needs so that he is distracted from the need to scratch?*

Critical reflections

This chapter has given an overview of the complexities of health, and explored how poor or suboptimal levels of health can impact on children's well-being. In the last 50 years children's health has become a complex area so an understanding of the child health policy is vital. More importantly, looking at historical developments in child health indicates that there is no room for complacency, especially when considering infectious diseases.

The critical questions should have helped you to unpack some of the issues in relation to education and promoting health. The overview of government child health policy contextualises the interventions that are topical and necessary in order to promote good health for all children and, in turn, increase their levels of well-being. The goal of promoting health and well-being demands a great deal from professionals, and one of the most important facets of being able to fulfil this aspect of an increasingly complex role is that you have an understanding of the key points about children's health and how you can contribute to children's well-being.

Critical questions

» *Carry out an audit of the health conditions, or health concerns, for the children in your setting.*

» *What interventions could you put in place to support their health?*

» *How could you change the environment, or support them to cope with the environment, in order to improve or maintain their health?*

» *What are the implications in relation to adapting the aims of the EYFS in order to develop inclusive practice for children with heath needs?*

Further reading

The following websites provide useful and up-to-date information relating to children's health issues.

DfE (Department for Education) (2013a) *Managing Medicines in Schools: Schools Activity Pack about Eczema*, www.education.gov.uk/schools/pupilsupport/pastoralcare/b0013771/managing-medicines/schools-activity-pack-about-eczema. Accessed 21 July 2013.

PHE (Public Health England) (2013a) *HPA: Health Protection Agency Homepage. Protecting People, Preventing Harm, Preparing for Threats*, www.hpa.org.uk. Accessed 21 July 2013.

Includes advice on preventing the spread of infection in schools and childcare settings available from:

PHE (Public Health England) (2013b) Vaccination Schedule, www.hpa.org.uk/web/HPAweb&Page&HPAwebAutoListDate/Page/1204031508623. Accessed 20 July 2013.

4 The social worker perspective

IAN LLOYD

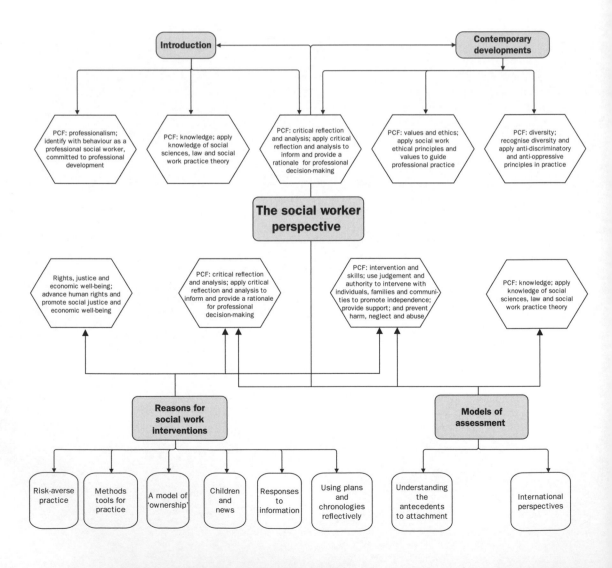

Introduction

Following the cessation of the General Social Care Council (GSCC) from 1 August 2012, the social work profession is now regulated in terms of professional membership, major disciplinary investigations, and education and training by the Health and Care Professions Council (HCPC). This organisation is not newly formed but evolved mainly in name from the Health Professionals Council, and has regulated the health professions for a number of years. In the advent of this development it has to be noted that the way in which social work students are educated and how the profession is regulated will be changed. The assessment of social work students in practice learning opportunities is also changing; this change sees the criteria to progress through the degree move from an actuarial process (tick-box of competency) to a holistic overview of capabilities. The visual map at the start of this chapter will guide you as to which aspects of the content are relevant to the 'professional capabilities framework'; this is the structure of progressive development that social work professionals are required to adhere to and follow in the course of progression and continuing professional development. More information and detail about these perspectives can be found at www.hcpc-uk.org (HCPC, 2013).

Social work has always been a service that stands alone, but is often misunderstood and confused with other services by professionals, the public and service users themselves. Prior to the 1970s some traditional social services had been undertaken by the local priesthoods, general professionals and the wives of upstanding and wealthy members of society. The formative development of the original 1954 legislation specific to social work with children resulted in the Adoption Act (1976); this was contemporary recognition regarding the need-levels of children who had been adopted, and indeed the welfare of parents whose children had been adopted. The dated Matrimonial Causes Act (1973) concerned the division of matrimonial assets following divorce, and fell very short of recognising the welfare of children and families involved in such marital breakdowns. The resulting impact on the welfare of children was recognised partly as a consequence of John Bowlby's development of attachment theory in 1957. Ironically, this was a psychological theory that has subsequently been adopted by the social work profession. However, as time has passed, the recognition of an independent and autonomous social service for children has been supported by legislation, such as the Children Act (1989), the Adoption and Children Act (2002), the Children Act (2004) and the Local Authority and Social Services Act (1970). Subsequently, and in response to the changing state or perspectives of society, many aspects of policy have responded to the needs of children and their welfare. The social work profession is constantly reminded of its involvement in serious case reviews, and as a result there has been a plethora of guidance to help orchestrate partnership and interprofessional working methods. The contemporary statutory guidance, *Working Together to Safeguard Children*, which came into effect in April 2013 (DfE, 2013b), updates the previous version from 2010. The assessment framework for the assessment of children in need and their families (2000), and the 2007 statutory guidance on making arrangements to safeguard and promote the welfare of children under section 11 of the Children Act (2004) remains effective and in place.

This chapter identifies the changing role of social work in a contemporary society, where the government wrestles with the challenge of a budget deficit; a changing society of people who use social services (Fox Harding, 1997); and the children and young people who are the future of this, our society. In doing so, it focuses on the well-being of the children who come into contact with social work.

Setting the scene

Since the early 1990s, there has been a significant development in the reliance on welfare budgets and the benefits system, and the necessity to monitor the welfare of children from all areas of society. The guidance previously referred to cites the overarching responsibility of all members of society to be aware of the welfare of our children. Independent sector agencies such as the National Society for the Prevention of Cruelty to Children (NSPCC) have rolled out initiatives including the *Full Stop* campaign, seen through media outlets for a considerable time during the 2000s. The increase in such factors as divorce rates, second and third marriages and the phenomenon of reconstructed families (two families coming together following divorce, separation or financial gains) has created a greater reliance on social service input to support the situation in which families find themselves (Daniel and Ivatts, 1998).

To this end, there has been a widening in the social class of society (ONS, 2013) that now engages with service interventions, whose members come to the attention of educational welfare officers and join contemporary clubs and organisations that support the average working family to enable the wage earners to earn that vital living. There is growing demand for after-school clubs, nursery places and extended families to support the arrangements of today's family, which is a far cry from the assumed norm, or perceived traditional form, of mum, dad, 2.4 children and 0.5 of a dog. It is therefore imperative that professionals, volunteers and managers of these organisations work and consult together to maintain the welfare of our children: society's children.

Contemporary developments

It is understandable that there is now a general acceptance that some families become 'professional benefit employees' – they are cited as families who remain reliant on the benefits system as their form of income, with little encouragement, opportunity or aptitude to rejoin the employment market. As recently as March 2013, David Cameron continued to defend his speech made in Liverpool in July 2010, where he introduced his ideological 'Big Society'. The question remains, however, is it working? The latest amendments to the benefits system, with the introduction of Universal Credits and the recently announced (March 2013) change to the Disability Living Allowance, which will become the Personal Independence Payment (GOV.UK, 2013), would suggest that the changes are being managed rather than being successful; they have not been welcomed by either the recipients or those responsible for 'picking up the pieces'.

This chapter therefore explores the differing approaches and contexts of contemporary social work practice, to enable practice to be inspired, fit for purpose and autonomous while remaining part of the wider multidisciplinary service required for you to become and remain a developing and effective professional.

Critical questions

»   *Is the protection of children only prolific in disadvantaged areas of society? Or is it simply assumed that children will be less well cared for just because they come from a poorer background?*

»   *The recent discussions about the development of the number of classes in British society identify that the social divides are 'widening'. Does this mean that children will have more opportunities for a safe and appropriate upbringing, or is it reflective of changes in dynamics, and therefore that there are fewer 'communities' to promote family and extended family?*

Reasons for social work interventions

It has to be recognised that there are continually evolving reasons for children to come into contact with social work interventions. The continued phenomenon of social drug use is becoming pandemic within society; it is high on the agenda of child protection professionals. The impact of drug use is far reaching, and is recognised as one of the most common causes of family disputes, breakdowns and social work interventions. The impact can be seen as twofold: service users who are experiencing problems with substances themselves, and those affected directly by another person's use of drugs. This second group typically includes partners, parents, siblings and children (Allan, 2010). You should of course give consideration to what is thought of as a 'drug'; the list is extensive and, as identified by Edwards (2005), refers to *mind acting* substances, including alcohol, tobacco, solvents and other volatile substances, and finally drugs. This includes all drugs, irrespective of whether they are identified as restricted under the Misuse of Drugs Act (1971). The impact of drugs on families is immeasurable, but Cohen and Kay (1994) demonstrate that society gives out and receives mixed messages about substance use and misuse. Media reporting dichotomises the issue. A death caused by ecstasy use is met with calls for law enforcement to apply rigorous action to tackle drug-dealing; a death caused by binge-drinking is met with calls for better public education – in the first instance the drug itself is seen as the problem, but in the second the issue with alcohol is considered one of irresponsible use.

While you can recognise and select a wide array of differing reasons for this societal problem, we as a profession need to take responsibility, with some points of good practice to ensure that we achieve the best for the service user group while operating with *defensible* rather than *defensive*, practice.

Risk-averse practice

During the course of their normal working day, social workers make decisions that have an impact on people's lives. Often they are operating with minimal information and are forced to make decisions within specific time frames. Many of the decisions they make involve dealing with significant risk and often have far reaching effects on the lives of individuals. It is therefore extremely important that the influences and the biases that affect these decision processes are better understood.

(Strachan and Tallant, 1996)

This quotation helps you to consider how to approach practice. It could be argued that a reflective professional should always consider that there is a risk – and one should look for evidence that will negate that risk or prove that it does not exist. To approach it from a *this is safe and I will look for the risk if it is there* angle places you, as a professional, on the back foot. It has to be recognised that service users and their families are not involved with social work as part of their general family life, but that the relationship is there because help, support or statutory support and interventions have been identified as needed by a wide range of professionals, and that the individual or their family has met qualifying criteria with a protection element characteristically attached. Not responding or practising accordingly could have deleterious outcomes. I will return to discuss the 'bias' in decision-making in the *Critical reflections* section found later in this chapter (pp 96–97).

Critical questions

» *What is risk to you? There are many concepts of risk, and the word itself may suggest urgency or immediacy. Social work sometimes deals with hidden risk that predates your involvement, so how do you justify identifying a perceived risk for someone who has managed that aspect of their lives so far without injury or harm?*

» *Is the management or identification of risk easier to categorise if we assess someone's reaction or perception of that risk, rather than simply identifying the risk itself? Might a risk to one person be a fact of life to another?*

Methods and tools for practice

In contemporary social work provision, targets, outcomes and resolutions are high on the agenda in identifying success (Aldgate, 2007). In order to get the best outcomes for service users, the children and their families' professionals will need to ensure they practise with scope, wide vision and accountability. The Department of Health (DH, 1996) reported the voice of children who stated that they are appreciative of workers who are their champions and who explain clearly what is going to happen, who also have the ability to stop and listen to the child's own side of the story or what their understanding of the situation is. All too many times you hear of children who have been placed, persuaded and 'managed' into situations that are not best suited to their needs but that tick a box or meet a target. The reality is that some social work practices fall far short of the needs of the children we are responsible for protecting. The research established overwhelmingly that in terms of a voice the child wants to be seen as a whole, not just as a child with problems (Rose, 2006).

John Bowlby established in 1953 that to meet the needs of children appropriately we need to cherish and support the parents (Bowlby, 1953); this in turn reflects on social workers, who cannot promote secure attachments in children if indeed the parents themselves are not supported and respected.

Planning for practice, intervention and outcomes will always give the professional a sense of direction, achievement and satisfaction at any given point throughout the course of their work.

Planning an intervention is always better than an intervention dictating what we do; this means that having a goal, a shared goal, will always give a better chance of success if it is owned and 'cherished' by all of those involved.

A model of 'ownership'

In terms of *reflection on* and *reflection in* practice (Schön, 1987), it has been identified that you respond better to a situation or a request to do something if you initially own it. For example, if something has happened that creates a problem for someone else, and they challenge you over it, if you do not believe or accept that you have some responsibility or ownership of the issue you may become defensive. If, however, you recognise that you had a part to play, it is less likely that the challenge will even be required, because you will act retro- spectively to make amends or immediately respond at the start of the challenge and agree a solution. This model can be rolled out in many ways. I first saw this approach to the model of ownership when I worked for a charity that searched for members of divided and separated families. As a social worker I was acutely aware that when meeting with a comparative stran- ger (an adult) to tell them they had a half-brother, half-sister or other half-relative, if I told them outright that they had this relative who wanted to get in touch I was in fact telling them that their family as they understood it was a lie: that perhaps their mother had been having an illicit affair or that the family had a dreadful and shocking secret. While it may have been a secret, what I was actually talking about was a member of their family. A practice tool that can be used to impart this knowledge without shock or rejection is a birth certificate. This simple tool – something that each and every one of us has – can simply be placed on the table and the person asked to tell you what it means to them. They will instinctively identify the people they know on the certificate: perhaps the name of their mother and the name of their father, or perhaps just the name of their mother, before, and perhaps with some encouragement, they begin to realise that the subject of the certificate is in fact related to them. They will work out that this person is then either their brother, sister, cousin, uncle or aunt. This means that they own the information for themselves rather than being told.

This model of approach maintains working relationships; it builds trust and creates a positive engagement. The news is generally accepted, and while it may be a shock it is usually owned and then cherished.

Likewise, as a professional you will always accept a criticism or challenge if you in the first instance accept or own the issue. Good managers or supervisors of social workers will dem- onstrate a perspective to be challenged, managed or dealt with; this in turn will be accepted by the professional, and thereby owned and dealt with more quickly than if the relationship is one of 'locking horns'.

Children and news

When you need or want to take children through change, they are likely to accept it better if they understand why the change has to happen rather than being pushed into it. Remember, with every change there is inevitably loss and gain. Piaget's cognitive theory helps us to rec- ognise points to remember when working with children in particular (Piaget, 1955).

Piaget's cognitive theory enables our own grasp of this to move beyond simply learning to active development, and to realise how children can develop their understanding and accep- tance. Piaget suggests that children can and will develop their understanding of a situation over time and, with the opportunity to reflect and reassert, will accept the information. Piaget breaks this down into three basic components:

1.   schemas – the building blocks of knowledge;

2.   assimilation and accommodation – the cognitive process of transition from one stage to another;

3.   stages of development – sensorimotor (birth–two years), preoperational (two–seven years), concrete operational (seven–ten years), formal operational (11+ years).

For this to become a working model, it will help to think of a set of building blocks. When the blocks are placed on a table in a wavy line, to a child it can become a snake or worm. When the blocks are placed on top of each other they can become a wall or shelf. When they are arranged in shapes they can become a box, a field in which to keep animals or a bed for their favourite teddy bear. This final shape can represent safety.

Lift one block out, and while on its own it is a block; it may be a part of something bigger, better or worse. The individual blocks (schemas) put together can tell a story.

This story becomes a part of the child and their understanding of the situation (assimilation and accommodation), and when they have sufficient blocks they will in their own unique way work out what it means. It is important to identify here that the child will work this out in their own way: not ours, not Piaget's, but their own. We provide the information in block-sized pieces; the child will build the wall, the box or the shape.

The age of the child and their ability to comprehend will always dictate the level of understanding. Moreover, children with additional disabilities will require further consideration in terms of their development, understanding and ability to process information in a world where they are perceived to be different (Hughes, 2012). For the younger child, the use of play therapy or acting will enable an age-appropriate understanding of the news they are receiving. Toys, books and items kept in a small box in your car will always help to tell the story; using items to relay information will edify to the child what it is you need to tell them. This is particularly effective if they have created the item, picture or model that represents the issue, and briefing the child's carer will allow reinforcement of the information at subsequent stages as they work out and accept the detail. Big news, changes and, in particular, loss cannot and should not be delivered in a short 15-minute visit on the way to another meeting or on the way home. This process takes time to prepare for, and it takes time for the child to accept the information. They may be angry (loss/fear), quiet (confused/scared) or appear to cope very well (denial/unwillingness to accept) when the news has been given.

Time to absorb, reflect upon and digest the news will need to be considered; for a child who experiences repeated loss, a place or area where the news is given will need to be away from a place they should associate with safety. Bad news given around the kitchen table with everyone present, or in their bedroom, can trigger unhappy feelings in the future, especially when all of the same people sit around the table – this could signify to the child that bad news is coming, and may explain why challenging behaviours are seen at such events as birthday parties.

Responses to information

Leon Festinger (1957) developed a theory about how we respond to information. This theoretical model helps us to identify when individuals may reject information because of physiological experience or lack of understanding. It is still a form of grief and loss theory.

Festinger identifies four stages that you go through when you learn something new, before you fully accept the information as part of what you do (*assimilation* (Piaget, 1955)). The four stages are as follows:

*   unconscious incompetence;

*   conscious incompetence;

*   conscious competence;

*   unconscious competence.

If you look at each, you can initially associate with the unconscious incompetence stage: you are not aware of what you do not know. Next, you are alerted to the fact that you do not know something: you become conscious of your 'incompetence'; but if you learn or absorb/accept the news or learning you then become aware (conscious competence) of what you have learnt or gained. Finally, when you fully accept the learning and it becomes part of everyday life, it becomes unconscious competence.

The classic example of this in practice is learning to drive. While you are learning to drive, you go through the repetitive motions: mirror, signal and manoeuvre. As you progress in your adeptness to assume this as an instinctive process and reaction you stop using the words, but do it automatically. How many times have you driven home, but then cannot recall the journey?

The less-acknowledged, but equally effective, application of this theoretical model is when you apply it to everyday life, learning and, in particular, change. The use of Festinger's theory in accepting change may enable us to understand where and why people reject that change or news; following the conscious incompetence part of the cycle, and before they move to the conscious competence stage, they may become afraid or threatened by the change because they do not know what it holds for them. This is where an individual may 'step off' the process, unwilling to accept the news, change or difference it brings about. One may retreat to an old position and refuse to accept the information, believing things can remain the same as they always have been. This is where you may see professionals trying to highlight the positives in this change, where what the child or individual may need is time to grieve for what has been or is about to be lost. There are a wide range of models of loss and grief (Payne et al., 1999; Currer, 2001; Hooyman and Kramer, 2006) and all will be relative to specific situations. While the cores of these are centred on bereavement, the models used can be applied with care to situational change where loss is experienced. One should never underestimate the impact of loss, particularly with children; this is most apparent where what may be a minor change to us as adults may be catastrophic to the child. The lack of understanding on our part about the relative grief in loss may represent to the child that you do not understand, care or take any responsibility for that change. Each and every one of us has the ability to be reactionary; likewise you also have an equal ability to adapt safely to change. The change that is most commonly rejected is one that is forced upon us by others.

Critical questions

»   *How can you measure the effect that change has on someone? A change in one person's life may not have the same impact on another. Does change only ever affect one person? Do you think other people with a positive attachment may be affected also?*

» *Do you think change will be more readily accepted if the ultimate goal or outcome is identified from the start? A good analogy of this is to imagine a car journey with strangers: without a map, any inkling of when it will start and finish, and not knowing destination. Does this make any sense? Is this the same as social work without a plan?*

Using plans and chronologies reflectively

Tools that can be effective in social work are plans or chronologies. These are essential tools in reviewing what has happened so far, and planning what to do next.

Planning for a change, particularly where that plan is built in collaboration with the subject of that plan, will always optimise the chances of success. This is indicative of the previous discussions about the model of ownership. Children in particular will absorb change better in the long term if they are part of the planning for that change. Behaviours or acting out may still be witnessed, but with the carers of that child fully briefed about the plan, and with play opportunities and models in place, the child will work through the stages of change (*development* (Piaget, 1955)) in a safer and better place.

A chronology of what has happened so far can sometimes, when reviewed reflectively, identify patterns, processes or issues that may not ordinarily have been seen when taken for granted.

CASE STUDY

Timothy's story

The following example of an excerpt from Timothy's case file that is offered to a prospective foster carer or adopter may demonstrate the point more effectively. The numbers in the example are referred to in the next section, *Bringing the information together* (pp 86–92).

Timothy (arrived 20.02.10) is a lively little boy (1) with an outgoing and bubbly personality. He eats ice cream with gusto, (2) and is constantly on the go. (3) Timothy enjoys new experiences, but does flit from one thing to another, (4) finding it difficult to concentrate on one thing for very long. (5) This is probably age-related and appropriate for his three years. When Timothy arrived with us, late one evening he clung to Marcia, the social worker, (6) for over an hour before being persuaded gradually to let go, when he then clung as keenly to me. (7) A little while after Marcia left, (8) Timothy gradually relaxed and played with some of the toys and had something to eat. Shortly after 7.30pm, he went to bed and settled almost immediately to sleep, (9) and slept for a solid 12 hours. The following morning, and after each night of at least 12 hours sleep, Timothy wakes to devour a hearty breakfast (10) before embarking on his days of adventure and exploring new opportunities. He loves riding his scooter, and wants to take it everywhere with him even when we go out in the car. (11)

For the two years he has been with us, (12) Timothy has enjoyed new experiences, and while his behaviour can at times be a little boisterous (13) he is readily distracted to another task. (14) Timothy is identified to have regular contact with his Mum, which she attends intermittently. (15) He takes this in his stride (16) and when he returns to the house he plays out on his scooter (11a) before eating his tea and going to bed for another of his famous mammoth sleeps. (9a) This is also the case after a nursery day, where he is well thought of even though he commands (17) control of the Lego box!

(Karen, Timothy's foster mother)

While, on the face of it, this looks very positive, if we then look at a chronology written by the social worker prior to the placement we see a different picture emerging from Timothy's perspective (Table 4).

Bringing the information together

The two excerpts of information provided in Karen's narrative and the social worker's chronology are scaled-down versions of what you would expect to be the real recording process. The foster carer has clearly done a very good job with Timothy, but if you interrogate the information more critically you can start to draw out some perspectives that may warrant further investigation or discussion.

If Timothy were to be moved to another foster carer, or indeed to an adoption placement, the above, combined with the chronology, might invite a series of critical questions.

Questions for you to consider

Below are some examples of questions that a social work professional might use to review what has happened so far. They are numbered to correspond to the numbered points in the case study above.

1. *Timothy is a lively little boy.*

    • What exactly does the foster carer mean by *lively*?

    • Is this liveliness constant, or is it a response to a structure or routine?

    • Structure or routine may not be something Timothy has experienced before.

2. *He eats ice cream with gusto.*

    • Does Timothy eat or devour his food? Is he constantly seeking food, or indeed stealing or hoarding food?

    • Is he ever sick after eating this food? Does he eat for the sake of it? Is he settled at mealtimes or does he appear 'hyper' or unsettled?

    • Is he willing to try new foods? Can he recognise the taste of food or tell you what it is?

3. *[Timothy] is constantly on the go.*

    • What are his behaviours like when he is doing this? Erratic? Is he in a world of his own?

    • Can he sit and concentrate on any tasks? Is he interested in TV? Does he use books, pictures or toys in imaginative play?

Table 4 *Timothy, and what happened preceding his arrival at the foster carer's*

23.04.09	Timothy John Dempsey born at Cancliffe Maternity Hospital.
24.04.09	Timothy made the subject of an initial assessment owing to ongoing concerns about previous drug use by his mother, Tracy John. Dad – Stuart Dempsey – is reportedly not on the scene. May be in prison?
26.04.09	Timothy's Apgar score recorded as abnormal; medical advice is for Timothy to remain in hospital for at least a week.
28.04.09	Discussion held with Louise John (Tracy's mum), who advises that Tracy still has contact with Stuart Dempsey. Tracy denies this.
03.05.09	Tracy reported as absent from the ward for over an hour. When she returns, she is reported to be elated and excitable. When challenged, she retorts that Timothy is safe; she needed some time out and met her friends for a coffee.
06.05.09	Timothy is making good progress, and a planning meeting with Tracy, Louise John and Cate Lewis (health visitor) agrees a discharge to the home of Louise John. She has agreed to take responsibility for overseeing Tracy and Timothy.
11.05.09	Out of hours (OOH) team record a call from a concerned neighbour reporting that Tracy was seen out in town late at night with Timothy. OOH social worker made contact with Louise John who assures them that Tracy is at the home asleep.
06.07.09	Three-month review – Timothy is making good progress; no report received from health visitor, and Louise John reports that everything is well and settled.
01.12.09	Call from health visitor to report that she has been off ill; on her return she tried to make contact with Tracy John. After speaking to Louise John she reports that Tracy has moved in with her friend in town – everything, including Timothy, is well.
03.12.09	General inquiries made in respect of Timothy's whereabouts. Some confusion, as neighbour reports that Timothy is regularly seen with Louise John (daily) and Tracy visits the house occasionally.
05.12.09	Report from health visitor to advise that Tracy has been in attendance at local police station with Stuart Dempsey: no charges, but warning for causing disturbances.
12.12.09	Home visit to Louise John, Timothy present and appearing to be well. Tracy reportedly returned to the home approx. 30 mins. after my arrival following a shopping trip.
04.02.10	Six-month review – Tracy arrived back at the house late, reporting she had a GP appointment that overran. Review was positive: Timothy making good progress and despite finding the extra responsibility tiring Louise reports she enjoys having Timothy and Tracy around.
07.02.10	Call from local police – Tracy remanded in custody with another adult, following arrest for reportedly dealing drugs.
09.02.10	Call from Louise John – she does not feel able to look after Timothy any more. The responsibility is not one she had bargained for and she feels uncomfortable with the visitors she receives looking for Tracy. Louise reports that Tracy has been staying away for longer periods over the last few months, so Louise feels used and compromised by the situation.
16.02.10	Search and contact with Karen Jones, foster carer, who can offer temporary accommodation to Timothy.

4.   *[Timothy] does flit from one thing to another.*

- What is his concentration like?
- Is Timothy aggressive with his change, can he be distracted or is his change a determined one?

5.   *[Timothy finds it] difficult to concentrate on one thing for very long.*

- Does he appear bored when he changes activity?
- What is his level of understanding in play?
- Does he act scenarios out?

6.   *[H]e clung to Marcia, the social worker.*

- Is this reaction normal? Is this a reaction to being moved, or a safety response to a changing environment? Can you ascertain if Timothy is used to different people? What is his attachment to his mother or grandmother like?
- Does Timothy make effective attachments? Can this be tested? Is hiding his face a safety mechanism?

7.   *[Timothy] clung as keenly to [Karen].*

- How does Timothy respond to change? He may see Marcia as the person responsible for that change and thereby feels safer when he is away from her?
- Has Timothy relaxed because he is used to going and staying at different people's houses?
- It may be worth noting that there was no mention of Timothy crying or sulking, which may be a more expected reaction in a child with a secure attachment?

8.   *A little while after Marcia left, Timothy gradually relaxed.*

- Has the threat of what Marcia represents gone? What has been the response or body language from Tracy and Louise when they have had contact with Marcia? Despite her acting in Timothy's best interests, may his awareness of other people's behaviour when she is around leave him thinking she is a bad person?
- Is Timothy used to a chaotic household? Does a settled, quiet and tidy house when Marcia is around feel wrong to him? Is Marcia the common denominator to this perspective?

9.   *[Timothy] went to bed and settled almost immediately to sleep.*

- While, on the face of it, this may appear to be very positive, has Timothy been used to long periods of time in his cot/bed? Does he 'hide' in sleep as a defence mechanism to feel safe? Has he listened to arguments, bustle and noises that may represent the lead-up to other events? His mum may have engaged in drunken or drug-influenced behaviour – might Timothy have learnt to find solace and safety in his cot, not daring to make a noise for fear of the reactions?

- Has Timothy learnt to stop crying for attention in the mornings? After learning that the response he receives if he makes demands is not a favourable one he may have coped by waiting to be woken up when 'they' are ready?

10.   *Timothy wakes to devour a hearty breakfast.*

- Does Timothy make the most of a square meal after having become used to surviving on intermittent meals, scraps of leftovers or even no food at all on some days?

- May Timothy steal food or eat it because it is there, rather than because he is hungry?

11.   *[Timothy] wants to take [his scooter] everywhere with him even when we go out in the car.*

- Does the scooter represent safety to Timothy? When an argument may have broken out, or if the house was full of people, he may have recognised that playing on his scooter in the garden kept him away from the people, arguments and trouble. Is he still doing this to feel safe, and as a distraction from all of the change that he does not understand?

- Does Timothy staying busy not come to the attention of his carers? Does his scooter represent play time with people but also time to be on his own? Perhaps he believes that riding his scooter may bring back some of the good experiences?

12.   *For the two years he has been with us ...*

- What has been the plan – why two years? Have there been any plans to reunite Timothy's family again? Have any other options, such as a family-and-friends placement or an adoption placement, been considered? Has any other placement been made – it could have only been recorded as contact. However, Timothy may have been given the messages of a potential home or a move?

- Each time the plans do not work out or fail, Timothy has got to re-engage with or attach to Karen. Does he feel that if he does certain things it means he gets to go back to Karen's again and avoid sadness?

13.   *[W]hile his behaviour can at times be a little boisterous ...*

- May Timothy have experienced rough-and-tumble play time, and is this the only way he knows to get a response (even if it is a negative response, it is a response)?

- Does gentle or caressing play represent the start of something that Timothy does not want to remember? Perhaps he remembers something he found physically painful or aggressive?

14.   *[H]e is readily distracted to another task.*

- Is this a survival tactic? Has he learnt to 'go with the flow' in a chaotic household to avoid conflict or arguments?

- Has Timothy learnt that crying to carry on playing with something may have incited a negative response? Learning to accept the move to something else could be another survival technique?

15. *Timothy is identified to have regular contact with his Mum, which she attends intermittently.*

- Is Timothy not disappointed because he does not expect her to be there?

- Does he not miss his mum when she is not there because he does not have a secure attachment to her?

- Timothy may have experienced some adults around him wanting to cuddle him when he is sad. May cuddles in the past have come to represent the start of something that hurt Timothy?

16. *He takes this in his stride.*

- Is this an adult perspective? Perhaps there is nothing to take in his stride?

- If Timothy has ambivalent or avoidant attachments is that why he does not feel the hurt that adults are expecting him to feel?

17. *[H]e commands control of the Lego box.*

- Is this an element of control for Timothy? Does he, in order to feel safe, seek control over the other children around him? As a professional, could you seek views about his response to both younger and older children – particularly if they are smaller than him – and to pets?

- Consider the aspects of his life that are out of his control. Is this one area, often unchecked, that he *can* control? Perhaps if he appears to play happily with the Lego he is left alone, but other children playing with him may disrupt that independence?

The two reports above are incomplete, but even from this limited information it is possible to create a series of questions that interrogate the scenario presented. Despite the willingness of the professionals and service users involved, and the expectation that the information you receive from them will be comprehensive, case load pressures and high work demands will sometimes result in an abridged version of information: one that characteristically falls short of its purpose.

If you also consider this case scenario in terms of existing knowledge using a tool such as a family tree or genogram, you can spot familial patterns that will help you to understand critically the nature of a pattern within a family and how this may impact learnt or developed behaviour. The concept here is not just to accept what you 'can see' but to interrogate what you 'cannot see'. (See *Models of assessment* later in this chapter (pp 93–96).)

The simple but effective genogram (Figure 7) can be used as a tool of reference, or to help with your assessment planning. Understanding the dynamics within a family is a value-based and constructive way of approaching assessment, care planning and outcome targets.

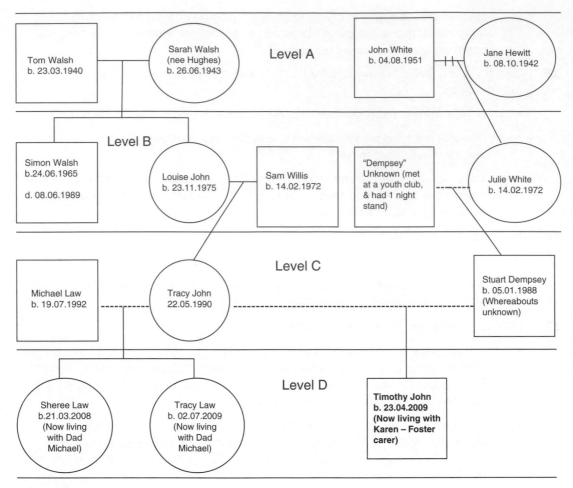

Figure 7 Timothy's genogram

Information

Level A

Tom and Sarah Walsh enjoyed a reasonably settled and happy marriage. Their first son, Simon (level B) was born with mild learning difficulties, and though he struggled at school he managed to gain employment on leaving, securing a job with a building firm. Simon tragically died in 1989 following a hit-and-run incident in the local town when he had gone to fetch his sister Louise home from a friend's house after missing her curfew time.

Their daughter, Louise John (level B), Timothy's grandmother, was a good school student, but shortly after her brother's death she became pregnant by Sam Willis (level B), a local youth known to some degree to the police.

John White and Jane Hewitt (level A) 'endured' a volatile relationship, attributable mostly to John's alcohol use. Jane had a series of jobs, most of which she either left unannounced or was dismissed from following a series of incidents with her partner John on work premises. They had one daughter, Julie (level B), who despite her academic ability rejected school, training and work; she favoured time with locals who worked intermittently on market stalls at weekends and market days. Julie met and had a sexual encounter with an unknown man known only as 'Dempsey'; she fell pregnant and had a son, Stuart Dempsey (level C). Stuart and his mother reportedly never saw 'Dempsey' again.

Level B

Louise John had a brief relationship with Sam Willis, who was already married and had a family. After a few months of living together on and off, they split up and Sam returned to his wife and children.

Level C

Tracy John met Michael Law while at school, and though they never married, they initially had a reasonably stable relationship. Tracy became pregnant at 15, and had a daughter, Sheree (level D) (b. 21.03.2008); she then became pregnant again and called her second daughter Tracy (level D) (b. 02.07.2009).

Shortly before her daughter, Tracy junior, was born, Tracy senior met Stuart Dempsey. They saw each other on and off, as Michael Law worked away from home to earn money, local work being very scarce and attracting only low pay. Shortly after Tracy junior was born, Tracy senior became pregnant again by Stuart Dempsey; this understandably caused major arguments with Michael when the relationship was discovered and made public on an internet chat site. The welfare of both Sheree and Tracy junior was questioned following volatile arguments at the flat. Shortly before Timothy's birth, Michael Law took his two children to live with him at his parents' house. Tracy senior agreed to this, and it was monitored by the local authority. They maintained their support for the arrangement because of their ongoing concerns relating to Stuart Dempsey, who at this point had already been in prison on two occasions, first for receiving stolen goods and second for actual bodily harm.

Despite high levels of support for Tracy senior, her ability to care for Timothy remained in question; what she reported and what was seen appeared at face value to be very different. This caused a high level of concern for Timothy's welfare.

If, as a professional, you consider all three perspectives – the foster carer's records, the social work chronology and finally the genogram – you will find that you are able to assess for and recognise the patterns, perspectives and issues that have potentially 'lived' through the families, and how they will have an impact on Timothy's outlook when it comes to his family, his future and how he feels about the people who, from a societal perspective, were supposed to protect and nurture him.

Critical questions

Consider Timothy's story.

» What impact do you think the loss of Simon Walsh had on his parents, his sister (Louise John) and, in turn, his niece (Tracy John)?

» Do you think that Tracy senior has any potential for ambivalent attachments following the death of her uncle, and the fact that she 'appears' to have readily relinquished her children, Sheree and Tracy junior?

» What do you think her feelings were when she met with Stuart Dempsey, who was born following an assignation between 'Dempsey' and his mother, Julie White, whose parents are described as having 'endured' a volatile relationship?

» Do you think Tracy would now feel abandoned (again) by Stuart Dempsey?

» What do you think has been Timothy's experience of security in terms of adults in his formative years? How readily will he be able to make secure attachments with subsequent adults?

To continue, you need to consider one of the most important skills in social work: assessment.

Models of assessment

The 'layered' model of assessment has a very simple approach: do not just assess what you can see, but look for what you cannot see. If you reconsider the approach to the earlier discussions about risk assessment (Chapter 1 by Strickland and Tallant in Kemshall and Pritchard, 2002) and apply the same perspective to the assessment and recording surrounding the case study of Timothy, you will in due course expose a systematic approach to the assessment. This in turn will deliver a report that is fit for purpose, and interrogates the information while guiding the reader or assessor to ask further questions in order to layer the detail. By considering the situation from differing perspectives it will give you a multidimensional picture rather than a 'one-sided' view.

Good practice would always indicate that a completed assessment is the start of the next step or process, both for the subsequent reader, and indeed in the outcome of the social work intervention for a child such as Timothy.

Modern-day social work demands sound assessment, and recognition of this as the basis for safeguarding and promoting the welfare of children (Aldgate, 2007).

In terms of the assessment of attachment, it is important to consider the issues raised in the introduction to this chapter (pp 78–79), where it was shown that contemporary society introduces substantially different challenges from those of the times when Bowlby (1953) and and later Ainsworth et al. (1978) developed their attachment theories. While social workers actively seek to assess levels of attachment, you may need to consider the effects and impact of the antecedents to attachment. For example, in Timothy's case study, what appeared at the first reading of his situation to be positive signs of attachment can, when looked at more closely (interrogated), begin to reveal other perspectives that should be considered and investigated for Timothy's welfare, future care and potential adoption. Aldgate et al. (2006) identify three fundamental principles in cases where children are separated from attachment figures.

•   Children react to the loss of their previous experiences of attachment

•   Children should be afforded the opportunity to express feelings of loss

•   Children will need sensitive and insightful care-giving to help them through the experience of loss

(Aldgate et al., 2006)

However, what may be less obvious is what to look for and how to identify where children have potentially not made a secure attachment. Issues and aspects of a child's life can be mistaken as a secure attachment. Take the example of Timothy: it can appear as though he is coping with his environment and relationships very well, and a variety of aspects within his life can be viewed as evidence that he has formed a secure attachment, when in fact the he may be displaying learnt survival behaviour as a coping mechanism or strategy. While Bowlby (1958), Howe (1995), Fahlberg (1994), Jewett (1984), Rutter (1985) and Daniel (2006), among many others, discuss the issues to look for in terms of children dealing with loss, what may need to be considered is that this is predominantly aimed at children with forming or formative attachments. In the case of Timothy, what appeared to be his coping with the change could in fact have been his 'blocking out' the experience; he may have been strategic in protecting himself.

Contemporaneously, you must be acutely aware of the child who has not formed an attachment. For example, a child like Timothy may have witnessed a violent relationship, or inadequate care pre- and post-birth; he may have been passed daily to different carers *just for a couple of hours*, or may have not had that nurturing time and opportunity to bond and form attached relationships with one particular person. Other reasons for Timothy's poor or non-existent attachments that could be identified as 'ambivalent' or 'avoidant' attachments include such diagnoses as Asperger's Syndrome, learning difficulties, autism and Foetal Alcohol Syndrome (FAS), among many other possibilities.

Timothy's reactions to his mother's lifestyle may also be indicated by his inability to form attachments, or his forming multiple shallow attachments rather than a strong attachment to one or perhaps two people. If Timothy's mother drank alcohol up to, during and following pregnancy, he may have been exposed to the risk of FAS. Foetal exposure to alcohol is one of the leading known causes of preventable intellectual disability (FASD Trust, 2013).

There is an extensive list of indicators for the child of a parent who has used or misused alcohol potentially to have Foetal Alcohol Spectrum Disorder (FASD), including:

•   learning difficulties;

•   problems with language;

•   lack of appropriate social boundaries (such as over-friendliness with strangers – can be mistaken for formative attachments);

•   poor short-term memory;

- inability to grasp instructions;
- failure to learn from the consequences of actions;
- egocentricity;
- mixing reality with fiction;
- difficulty with group social interaction;
- poor problem-solving and planning;
- poor co-ordination.

Research by the professionals at the FASD Trust suggests that, diagnosed early, FASD can be well managed. Advice to parents and teachers may be as simple as repeating instructions or allowing more time for tasks and learning opportunities. Further research, where a sample of adults with untreated FASD were assessed, found that 94 per cent had mental health problems and 64 per cent found themselves in the criminal justice system (Abel and Sokol, 1987).

In terms of the assessment of children like Timothy, who may come from such a background and are being prepared for long-term fostering or even adoption, the social worker must be aware and take account of the potential for this condition or symptoms to be present. Typically, where children with FASD are ambivalent in terms of attachment, the results, particularly for adoption, can be catastrophic and heart-breaking.

Understanding the antecedents to attachment

There are four generally accepted perspectives associated with attachment; the classification of these perspectives was initially suggested by Ainsworth et al. (1978) and subsequently developed further by Howe (1995, 2001).

- *Secure attachment patterns*. The child experiences their caregiver as available and also see positivity in their demeanour. Caregivers who are positive about themselves will engage with children and create an atmosphere of positive thinking, demonstrating to the child that all is good with the world.

- *Ambivalent patterns*. The child may experience their caregiver as inconsistent in their response, sometimes positive and frequently negative or withdrawn. The caregiver may themselves present as dependent and poorly valued, or with low self-esteem.

- *Avoidant patterns*. The child experiences continual rejection from their caregiver, possibly through being passed frequently to other carers. Especially when the child seeks affection and reassurance, the caregiver themselves presents as needy, insecure and compulsively self-reliant. The caregiver will be unable to reassure the child when they seek reassurance for themselves.

- *Disorganised patterns*. Associations can be made with children who have suffered severe maltreatment, cruelty or unnecessary punishment. Children see their caregivers as frightening, or indeed frightened, and simultaneously see themselves as helpless, angry and unworthy.

Critical questions

»   *Can you identify your attachments? In an emergency whom would you get in touch with? Whom would you talk to about a difficult decision? Are the people you choose to talk with about one decision the same as those for a different type of decision? Why is this?*

»   *Is it always a particular parent to whom a child will have an attachment? Is it possible that some children will have a better attachment to extended family rather than to their own mum or dad? Is this a problem? Would it change your opinion of the parent and their parenting style?*

INTERNATIONAL PERSPECTIVES

With increasing cultural diversity, the professional will need to be aware of cultural differences applicable to a diverse case workload of children from families in transition, in immigration or in search of a home following the persecutions of war and conflict.

Children settling in a new country when they have fled from all that they know and lost attachments of nuclear or wider familial life will respond very differently and uniquely. It is beyond the scope of this chapter to pursue each and every cultural difference of our modern world, but there is the opportunity for professionals to reflect upon their duty and responsibility critically to investigate the cultural perspectives of working with international families.

Van Ijzendoorn and Sagi have studied patterns of attachment across a wide range of cultures and countries, and state the following:

> *Not only has the attachment phenomenon itself but also the different types of attachment appeared to be present in various western and non-western cultures. Avoidant, secure and resistant attachments have been observed in the African, Chinese and Japanese studies; even in the extremely diverging child-rearing context of the Israeli kibbutzim, the differentiation between secure and insecure attachments could be made.*
>
> (van Ijzendoorn and Sagi, 1999, p 728)

Summary

One of the most critical aspects of good social work practice is the skill and art of reflection. A model of reflection will enable you as a professional to reflect on your practice and identify where you could improve your practice or try a different approach, but also of fundamental importance is that it will enable you to identify issues, problems and difficulties using information and perspectives that are given to you by fellow professionals.

The most important reflections are those that revisit the most difficult decisions you make. Brian Taylor discusses *decisions in crisis* and *emotion in decisions* (2010, p 20). He suggests that social work decisions are often made in crisis, with limited information and regularly against the wishes of the subject of that decision or, indeed, of close relatives or interested parties. Earlier in this chapter (*Reasons for social work interventions*, pp 80–86) I discussed *defensible* decision-making over *defensive* decision-making, and with each decision you make for and on behalf of other people in social work there is a high likelihood that there will be an element of vulnerability in the situations facing children and their families. You need to use models, plans and criteria in order to justify and defend the decisions you make. Janis and Mann present four simple and basic questions that you can use to help reflect on the decisions both before and after you make them.

1. Are the risks serious if I do not change?

2. Are the risks serious if I do change?

3. Is it realistic to hope to find a better solution?

4. Is there time to search and deliberate?

(Janis and Mann, 1977)

Deep analysis of your own ability to make decisions will, if considered carefully, enable you to identify the criteria you use to make those decisions. Are you influenced by other professionals you work with? Are you reluctant to see the perspective of the person you are making the decision about? Do you find it difficult to justify a decision that goes against 'the grain' or 'the tide' of everyone else around you?

The increasing pace of contemporary social work dictates that decisions will need to be made quickly, and often with limited information. There are similarities here to the Kemshall and Pritchard (2002) quote in the *Models of Assessment* (above, pp 93–96) section, where I discussed the challenges faced when making decisions about risk and risk factors. In both of these circumstances you may be influenced by 'bias' to determine or justify your decisions. You need to be aware of this bias to ensure that you do not make ill-thought-out decisions over specific and fit-for-purpose ones. Examples of bias in decisions are also seen in Strachan and Tallant (1995) where they offer the following suggestions in terms of what may influence your decisions.

*   *Representative bias*. This is the comparison of other experiences that are similar to or representative of the situation being observed.

*   *Availability bias*. This is the connection of an experience to available information; it can mislead a decision-maker towards conclusions based on information that has little bearing on the facts of the decision or assessment in hand. For example, the news headline *350 people die in air crash* might increase anxiety that plane travel is dangerous; it is in fact the safest form of travel.

*   *Confirmation bias*. This is the use of statistics to endorse the assessment or decision, where they may have no true relationship to the presenting facts.

A decision made where time is limited may be designed temporarily to reduce the immediate risk by 'holding' a situation for a period of time. Review and reflections on this decision may take the future case work in another direction: one that may aid recovery and repair where this is applicable. Over time you will, as a professional, use previous knowledge and 'bias' to help inform such decisions; experience will enable you to be more analytical in your approach and in the reasoning behind your decisions (Taylor, 2010).

Critical reflections

Analogies have been drawn throughout this chapter to help you consider your own development in terms of assessment practice and the reasons for social work interventions. This has been done while recognising the welfare of and focus on children who are in contact with social work. The development of such heuristics in practice is an important feature of the social work profession (Taylor, 2010), and in consideration of modern change the chapter focused on aspects of why society is an ever changing phenomenon. The children who are the recipients of developing social work practice need to be cared for by professionals who are reflective, developmental and secure in their ability to make sound decisions, and who are committed to good social work practice. To this end, the chapter examined risk-averse practice, and methods and practice tools that can help you as a professional to plan, progress and then review social work interventions. A model of ownership was introduced, to help you explore some of the challenges you face as a professional when planning methods of giving news and acknowledging the impact of such news on the recipients, particularly children.

The chapter looked at responses to information and how, by using plans, chronologies and genograms reflectively, you can see a 'bigger picture' that will help you reconcile behaviours, attitudes and responses to social work interventions. This approach can help with models of assessment. A thorough assessment process may help you not only to assess what you can see, but also to question critically and ascertain what you initially cannot see. The exploration of attachment and the antecedents to attachment are seen within international perspectives to help awareness of cultural differences within each and every society.

Further reading

McLeod, A. (2008) *Listening to Children: A Practitioner's Guide*. London: Jessica Kingsley.

Alison McLeod presents some excellent perspectives on and approaches to listening to children. Chapter 1 introduces you to the reasons why we should listen to children; Chapter 4 gives you some insight into how children develop ideas and concepts, and how they absorb information.

O'Loughlin, M; O'Loughlin, S. (eds) (2012) *Social Work with Children and Families*. 3rd edn. Exeter Learning Matters.

I have already referred to O'Loughlin and O'Loughlin, and Chapter 7 will guide you through the intricate processes involved in preparing children for change, foster care or adoption. While the process can be viewed as acutely actuarial and systematically driven, your practice in terms of the welfare of the child does not need to be. This chapter will introduce you to some of the reasons for the processes, and help you to understand them in terms of your work as a professional to help the child cope more readily.

Currer, C. (2001) *Responding to Grief: Dying, Bereavement and Social Care*. Basingstoke: Palgrave.

Caroline Currer will continue to help you develop concepts of loss and grief; more than just bereavement, grief is a multifaceted and complex process that children are not always able to articulate. Chapter 5 will help you with some guidance on effective practice in response to loss and grief.

Taylor, B.J. (2010) *Professional Decision Making in Social Work*. Exeter: Learning Matters.

Further to my reference to defensible practice over defensive practice, Brian Taylor will help you to explore professional judgement and how to use bias and knowledge to develop such defensible decisions in your practice. Decision-making in social work is one of the most challenging aspects; decisions are often made against the wishes of the subject of that decision. Where there are statutory and legal systems in place to help you, the emotive aspect is no less apparent. Where there are no statutes to enforce the decisions, you need robust and defensible systems in place to give you the confidence to practise defensibly.

Teater, B. (2010) *An Introduction to Applying Social Work Theories and Methods*. Maidenhead: Open University Press.

Barbra Teater provides excellent opportunity to develop your understanding of linking theory to practice; she will help you build a comprehensive understanding of how theory informs decision-making and the value base of your decisions. Teater revisits some of the perspectives of theoretical practice in social work, and guides you through the plethora of opportunities to interrogate your own thinking and approach to planning for outcomes.

5 The early years professional perspective: men in childcare

SUE CHAMBERS AND JUNE O'SULLIVAN

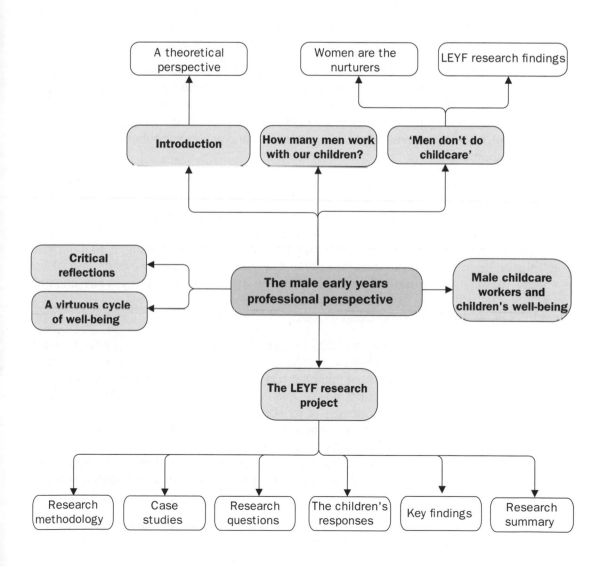

Introduction

It is surely a truism that those professionals who work with children want to contribute to their childhood by giving them a happy and fulfilled experience while in their care – an experience that will boost their talents and potential. Plato said that *the most important part of education is proper training in the nursery*, and more recently, in 2011, UNICEF noted that:

> [the] earliest years are one of the most critical times in human development and our investment here establishes the foundations of all learning in the future. There are sufficient data to support the positive potential of quality media that [are] age-appropriate during the preschool years to help prepare children for entry to school, while also supporting social, emotional, cognitive and physical development.
> (Kolucki and Lemish, 2011, p 17)

One way we make this investment is by using our roles as educators to understand and support children's well-being, which, according to an emerging consensus, is multidimensional and includes physical, emotional and social well-being, as well as children's beliefs and attitudes about themselves, their place in the world and their future life.

This chapter looks specifically at how having male staff in Nurseries can support children's well-being. It refers to ongoing research carried out by the London Early Years Foundation (LEYF) with the express aim of promoting the importance of male educators. The research findings offer concrete evidence that gender-balanced settings are not only good for children and staff alike, but also necessary for the improvement and advancement of children's learning and development.

LEYF began to consider how, as an organisation, it could best support the well-being of its male staff, with the intention of helping them to have the very best relationships with children and their families, and to improve the overall impact of their role in the settings where they were deployed. In addition, given the gradual shift towards engaging children and young people in the process of understanding what constitutes well-being, it was decided to ask the children for their perspective so that they could share their views as part of the research. This seemed particularly pertinent given the important differences in how children and adults view and define well-being (Davis-Kean and Sandler, 2001; Zaff and Hair, 2003; Sixsmith et al., 2007; Layard and Dunn, 2009).

According to Davis-Kean and Sandler (2001), access to appropriate enabling environments provides the support that is necessary if a child is to thrive. For them, key influencing contexts of young children's development included relationships, interactions and experiences at home, in childcare and in their community. Research by Fattore et al. (2007, 2009) concluded that the three overriding concepts of well-being as defined by children were a positive sense of self, security and agency. Emotional and relational well-being were integral to these concepts. This conceptual framework, characterised by the LEYF research, became the architecture of the process to find out directly from the children just how they defined their own well-being, and how the male professionals played a part in their feelings of happiness, security and well-being.

Well-being can be understood as a global state encapsulating all the elements that foster children's current and future health and happiness.

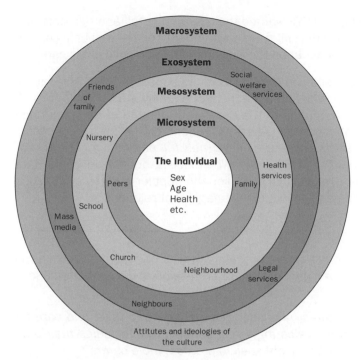

Figure 8 Bronfenbrenner's ecological systems model

A theoretical perspective

Bronfenbrenner (1979) and his *ecological systems theory* can be used to highlight the importance of the role of the nursery in a child's life. He describes the environment as *a set of nested structures, each inside the next, like a set of Russian dolls* (p 22). The developing child is at the centre of, and in fact embedded into, several environmental systems, from immediate settings such as home and family (the microsystem), to broader contexts such as school (the mesosytem). It is the interaction between these systems (or settings) illustrated in Figure 8 that shows the interconnectedness of children's lives internally and externally.

Oberhuemer et al. (2010) reaffirm this through their work, which shows the power that historical, cultural, economic and geopolitical contexts have on our views about who should work with young children. The well-being of staff also has a reciprocal benefit on the well-being of children. For example, Aeltermann et al. (2007) note that *Well-being expresses a positive emotional state, which is the result of harmony between the sum of specific environmental factors on the one hand, and the personal needs and expectations of teachers on the other hand* (p 286).

More recently, research led by the University of London supported the premise of a virtuous cycle of well-being (Briner and Dewberry, 2007). This research found that where teachers were significantly and positively engaged and had higher than average levels of job stimulation and enjoyment, school performance also improved. Put plainly, happier, motivated teachers could make children feel happier, motivated and more confident – although they found too that what goes up can also come down, and that poor staff well-being leads to demotivated staff, and thus to decreased well-being in children.

In addition to hearing from the children, LEYF wanted the research to tell another story: the story of the male professional working in the childcare environment and the well-being of that professional, which would no doubt impact upon the well-being of each child in his care.

It is logical to suppose that a gender-balanced workplace would benefit all staff. This rationale is supported by Veenhoven (2012), who found that gender equality is a key factor in self-reported well-being and happiness. According to the Chartered Institute of Personnel and Development, well-being at work is about *creating an environment to promote a state of contentment which allows employees to flourish and achieve their full potential for the benefit of themselves and their organisation*. The NHS Healthy Workplace Handbook advocates that a healthy gender-balanced workplace results in a healthier and happier workforce with good staff retention, low sickness absence and good staff–management relations.

Critical questions

» *There are many other professions that are predominantly of one gender. How do you evaluate your own perceptions of a gender-specific profession and a gender-balanced profession?*

» *For centuries, international cultures have used female carers to raise and care for offspring, often in groups of females caring for all the children, including their own. Can you think why western countries might seek to promote male carers?*

» *Consider well-being in terms of your role in childcare, teaching, role-modelling and as part of your own career. What does well-being mean to you?*

How many men work with our children?

The London Early Years Foundation conducted primary research among its own staff and children to ascertain an understanding of a gender-balanced workforce, and set it within a context of broader secondary research about male childcarers. Three key questions were asked:

1. What do people say about men working in childcare?
2. Does having male childcare staff benefit children's well-being?
3. How do we support male staff well-being so we can build a virtuous cycle of well-being?

These questions were investigated using an action–research approach, where we were asking questions and exploring how things could be improved to give children the best care and the very best staff – an approach sometimes described as look, think and act.

The number of men in childcare remains low, despite a number of government initiatives to increase it. The European Union set a target in 1995 to raise the proportion of men to 20 per cent, and by 2006 it had failed to happen. The Care Work in Europe project said that it was imperative to overcome the notion that care work is *what women naturally do*, and actively to address the gender gap in the ECEC workforce. The European Commission noted *an almost complete absence of men in the profession, reinforcing the stereotype that childcare is women's work only*, and *denying many children male role models*, and stated its intention to raise professional standards, increase levels of training and remuneration,

Table 5 *Men in childcare within Europe*

Country	% of men working in childcare	Year evidence collected
Norway	10	2008
Denmark	8	2005
Germany	3.5	2012
UK	2	2012
Netherlands	1–2	2008
Ireland	<1	2013
Austria	0.8	2006
Spain	Virtually 0	2013
Hungary	Virtually 0	2013
Russia	0	2013

improve the quality and motivation of the workforce, increase the number of male workers, and remove stereotyping (Cameron and Moss, 2004).

The UK coalition government pledged its support for a greater gender balance in the early years workforce, and Professor Cathy Nutbrown's review of early education commented on the low numbers of men working in the sector, believing this to be *about widespread social perceptions of what it is to work with young children and the widely held belief that this is 'women's work'* (Nutbrown, 2012). She voiced her belief that young children benefit from spending time with men as well as women. She recommended that, through the establishment of clearer career routes and an improvement to the perceived status of the early years workforce, more men will see the value of the profession, and be encouraged to consider working with children. However, despite such good intentions there are just 2 per cent in full day-care and childminding, and 1 per cent in sessional care across the UK. It is interesting to examine a graphical representation of the numbers across the world (Tables 5 and 6).

Critical question

»   *What do you think are the reasons for so few men working in the early years childcare sector? Are these historical reasons or are there justifiable reasons for men choosing not to work with young children?*

'Men don't do childcare'

Changing attitudes and beliefs takes time. Remember that each individual needs to change at their own pace. The overall message is one of valuing each individual for the skills and background they have. This includes their family background, race, beliefs, language and so on. Each individual sees the world through their own perspectives and with assistance through the perspectives of others.

(Arthur, 1993)

Table 6 Men in childcare across the world

Country/region	% of men working in childcare	Year evidence collected
United States	2	2007
New Zealand	2	2006
Australia	1.6	2006
Africa	Virtually 0	2013
South America	Virtually 0	2013
Asia	Virtually 0	2013

While there appear to be several reasons for the limited number of men in childcare, the most robust objection to men in childcare appears to be about how men are perceived within society. Cameron (2001) and Cameron and Moss (1999) believed the main reason for the predominantly female workforce in early childcare and education is that it is seen as *women's work*, and this reproduces its own patterns in recruitment and training.

> *It has had an impact on the historical and pedagogical understandings of why child-care exists, how it is conducted and organized, and what is gender appropriate have evolved through practice and policy over time.*

(p 8)

The Major Provider Group *Men in Childcare Report* (2011) polled 132 male school leavers aged between 16 and 19, 17 unemployed men and 39 male early years practitioners. Of the school leavers, 54 per cent said they would not want to work in a predominantly female environment and would feel social isolation; 50 per cent were worried about what other people would think. This included peer pressure and men's fears of being accused of inappropriate behaviour. They also voiced concerns about negative parent attitudes to men carrying out intimate care of young children; men felt they had to work much harder than women to gain parental trust. Concerns were expressed that there might be deep-rooted prejudices from women opposed to men working in childcare, that they would be expected to engage in stereotypical activities such as football and lifting heavy objects, and about the pressure of being a role model to young children. Of the respondents, 38 per cent cited low pay and status. They commented that the breadwinner needs higher earnings, and that the part-time nature of much childcare work better suits women, who need to fit work around their own childcare responsibilities.

Women are the nurturers

The work of Blount (2005), Fifield and Swain (2002) and Weems (1999) concluded that whereas women are viewed as nurturers, there is an assumption that men wishing to work in this context are often effeminate, homosexual and/or paedophiles. As a consequence, Farquhar et al. (2006) and King (1998) asserted that both homosexual and heterosexual men were discouraged from wanting to work with young children, further reducing the presence of men in early childhood education. Seifert (1988, 38, 69–80) believed that this stereotyping of men, implying that they are unsuitable to carry out a nurturing role, has made it difficult to recruit men into careers teaching young children.

Haase (2008) commented that *male teachers are also under a cloud of suspicion as to why they would choose primary teaching and would want to work with women and children*. Sanders (2002) suggested that male early-childhood teachers have to defend their choice of a profession to family, friends and female teachers – a comment also noted by all three men interviewed for this chapter (see below, pp 107–109). In the workplace, Murray (1996) found that *in the childcare environment men are often sought after as workers because of the perceived need to have male role models for children*, models that are seen as *doing truck play with the boys* (p 374).

Farquhar (2012) asserted that, as men are rare in early-childhood work, their employers and colleagues tend to regard them as something to brag about and show off as if they are a trophy or prized asset. She notes that while some men may find this attention amusing and flattering, there is also a negative side to being one of a few men in what is generally perceived as a woman's job. Again, this was noted by those men interviewed, and it was also a common theme in discussions at the London Network of Men in Childcare.

It is therefore not surprising that with one comment an article in *Nursery World* summed up the resistance as *I'm a man. And men don't look after children* (Morton, 2011).

Even more recently, a story reported in the *Mail Online* (14 September 2012) affirmed many of society's perceptions about stereotyping, not least with the introduction to an article about a male nanny:

> *It's normally only women who are trained in the art of turning curtains into costumes and become a dab hand at changing nappies at a world-famous nanny college. But now one male teenager is set to be the first-ever man to pass through the education degree course that turns out the modern Mary Poppins.*
>
> (Edwards, 2012)

Another factor that men at the London Network commented on was the feeling of isolation and *token male syndrome*. Farquhar (2012) had picked this up in her research, also reflecting on the feeling of isolation men can have in a female-dominated workplace with no male colleagues. In additon there was the burden of being under constant pressure to prove they were just as good as women at caring-type jobs, and being singled out for attention or being made to feel uncomfortable or different in an all-female environment. In a *Nursery World* article, a practitioner said *Being expected to assemble office furniture, move desks around, or to welcome being handed the office toolkit, are taken as read*. He went on to complain that as a man he was expected to fix the nursery computer because it was assumed that, as a man, he was an expert in IT (Anon., 2012).

London Early Years Foundation research findings

The LEYF research was noteworthy, in that 60.7 per cent of respondents felt the main reason for the low numbers of men in childcare was that men were not encouraged to join the profession, including by school and family, while another 51.8 per cent thought that it was because of society's attitude. In the Major Provider Group survey, 38 per cent thought poor pay and career structure were among the main deterrents, but this was not the key issue for the LEYF respondents, who scored 28.6 per cent and 12.5 per cent on these issues respectively. The comments from LEYF practitioners noted the apparent lack of advertising and a lack of awareness of what the job involves: particularly the responsibility for the education of the children.

> *For at least a year we ran a nursery where the majority were male and there were times when all the men were on duty. We experienced comments by tradesmen or the postman who expressed surprise more than objection.*
>
> (David Stevens, nursery manager)

The challenges are therefore widespread, and while there is also a great deal of support, it is clear that if we are encouraging men into childcare, we need to create a space for them that is welcoming and inclusive, and ensures that the message about gender-balanced workplaces are shared by both male and female staff.

A quote from a male colleague speaking at a conference in Helsinki in 2006 sums up the point when he says:

> *[I]n health, as in other social domains, the biggest challenge is perhaps to account more accurately gender as an ideology that interprets and gives meaning to men and women social role, ascribe behavioural patterns and promote inequality, inequity and power asymmetries.*
>
> (Vasco Prazeres)

Critical questions

» *What are the key benefits to children of men working in the early years sector?*

» *In what way does a male professional impact on children's learning?*

» *How is gender identity in a female-dominated environment different from that in a gender-neutral environment?*

Male childcare workers and children's well-being

> *Gender imbalances can be problematic in education, a field in which role modelling of diversity is crucial for pupils to be able to envision career possibilities that defy traditional identity norms.*
>
> (Gosse and Facchinetti, 2012)

The LEYF data is useful in highlighting some key issues surrounding male staff and their relationship with the well-being of children. It shows that all practitioners were in favour of men in childcare, but that there was generally a gross overestimation of the percentage of men working in the early years childcare sector, with only 10.7 per cent correctly estimating the figure at 2 per cent.

> *Mum and the maternal family were very supportive but Dad says it's a downgrade and it's not masculine. He respects that I have a job and I have to live with it. I've had lots of banter from Dad's family.*
>
> (Bryan Mansiamina, LEYF Apprentice)

When considering the benefits of men working in childcare, 75.0 per cent of LEYF practitioners believed it was very important for men to be seen as nurturing and sensitive role models, and another 50.0 per cent felt they could challenge society's attitudes towards men working with children. However, one of the main arguments for encouraging men into working in childcare is the importance of having both men and women in caring roles. Ruxton (1992, p 25) noted that the vast majority of early years staff recognised the importance of positive male role models for children and families that help to challenge the stereotypical view of men as *breadwinners* alone, and to validate their role as *carers*. Chodorow (1978) and Johnson (2008) pointed out that if most of our Nurseries are staffed by women, young children may make stereotypical assumptions about male and female roles. This reinforces notions about gender attributes and roles. Piburn (2006) noted that if more men were employed in childcare we would actively discourage these ideas of stereotyping, many of which are embedded in social culture.

Jensen (1998, p 122) made the case for a *gender pedagogy* and not a *gender-neutral* culture. He noted that boys and girls are different in some ways, and choose different games and activities. This presents different challenges to those employed, both female and male. He asserted that the daily pedagogic work must take these differences into account. He believed this can be more easily fulfilled by a mixed-gender workforce that will contain a greater diversity of masculine and feminine traits.

Johnson (2008) believed that caring for and teaching young children were appropriate and necessary roles for women and men. He said:

> Not only are gender stereotypes artificial, but they also can interfere with children's learning about interpersonal relationships, caregiver interdependence, and caregiving skills that all children need as they mature.

Cameron (2007) talked about a male worker who said he was conscious of reacting against performing in a stereotyped 'male' way:

> [I am] aware of situations where men have functioned in a completely different way with children ... when they're out in the garden, it's the men that are kicking the ball about and running up and down with it ... and I've consciously tried to prevent myself getting sucked into that.

In terms of play type, Fagan (1996), Parke (1996) and Lamb (2000) contended that men bring more active movement, entertainment, and rough-and-tumble play to the way they interact with their own children and the way they interact with children in general. They asserted that men do this, and encourage children to take more risks, because of their physical strength. Just recently, the European Parliament Committee on Women's Rights and Gender Equality (2012, p 5) commented that *Gender stereotypes in primary and secondary schools influence the perception of young children and youngsters of how men and women should behave.*

Given the current opinion that many children, especially of pre-secondary school age, lack a male role model in their life, and that many more have limited contact with fathers working long hours, it is not unreasonable to make the leap that both boys and girls can benefit from contact with positive male role models in early years and primary school contexts. Shonkoff and Phillips (2000) added to this with their research arguing that children's development is the result of the interaction between biological maturation and the environment, including their experiences and relationships. The basic architecture of the brain, which underpins all developmental domains, is built through an ongoing process that begins before birth, remains active during the early years and continues into adult life. Thus, having both men and women available to form relationships with children is a positive benefit.

Parents seem quite comfortable with this view, and Owen's (2003) studies of parental attitudes to men in childcare found that one clear reason why parents supported men working with young children was *concern for the boys*. He cited the example of a mother of a six-month-old boy, who said she was keen for there to be a male role model and felt strongly there should be a male contact for him as he got older. The British public is also broadly in favour of men working within the childcare profession, according to research from MORI in 2003. Three-quarters (77 per cent) were in favour and 12 per cent against. Many also recognised the benefits it can bring, particularly in providing positive male role models (mentioned by 53 per cent) and a mixed-gender environment (mentioned by 57 per cent).

> *Parents tend to see the benefit of a young role model setting good examples. I notice that dads come and chat to me unprovoked and say quite publicly they believe in what I am doing. With my age and all the negative stereotypes about young people it's very heartening to get positive feedback.*
>
> (Bryan Mansiamina, LEYF Apprentice)

More recently, Major Provider Group (2011) noted that almost all (97.8 per cent) of female childcarers in day Nurseries said they would value having male childcarers working alongside them as part of their team. Interestingly, 97.9 per cent of parents who use group childcare are happy for men to work with children aged three to five in day Nurseries. Parents felt men were more likely to play football, to do things outside and to *muck about*. They *let the kids get on with it* and *are not inhibited by risk*. Women, on the other hand, were seen by parents as providing the substantive, consistent parts of caring. He noted that parents reflected the observation that men in the home do the *fun* childcare and women do the routine nurturing.

Jensen (1998, p 122) asserted that since boys and girls are different in some ways, and choose different games and activities, they give different challenges to those employed; both female and male should be striving for a *gender pedagogy* and not a *gender-neutral* culture. He believed that the daily pedagogic work must take these differences into account and that this can be more easily fulfilled by a mixed-gender workforce.

The London Early Years Foundation research project

> *One of the most powerful lessons that I have learned is that even young children are able to reflect on issues that impact on their identity and their lives. The world of children is governed by the same values and beliefs that govern the world of adults*
>
> (Segura-Mora, 2002)

The London Early Years Foundation approached their research with the children using the principles set out by Dahlberg et al. (1999, p 49), who say that listening to children is about acknowledging that *children have a voice of their own, and should be listened to as a means of taking them seriously.* The Foundation looked at how research is undertaken with under-fives and found that few studies have addressed any research questions directly to the children. Sayeed and Guerin (2000, p 2) note that:

> research is largely based on observations of players (children) and non-players (adults) as the players are not generally expected to be able to describe what they are/were doing while they are/were engaging in play.

The London Early Years Foundation were aware that interviewing very young children as part of a research project is difficult for two main reasons. First, children's skills in reading and writing are not developed, and this constrains the possibilities of research methods. Second, their lack of maturity for understanding some types of questions and the difficulty of verbal expression also lead to very poor data-gathering.

The Foundation decided to use a model suggested by Clark (2000), using *mapping and modelling, diagrams, drawing and collage, child to child interviewing and drama and poetry*. Clark believed that these participatory research methods had particular relevance when seeking to reveal the multiple perspectives of young children. *who are themselves the least powerful individuals in the institutions they are part of* (p 3). Kuhn and Eischen (1997) and the Mosaic Approach cited in Clark and Moss (2001) also recommended that researchers present children with visual-based concepts rather than verbal statements in order to provide them with a framework that they can process and through which they can begin to provide feedback.

Using a methodology that was child-focused, LEYF conducted research across the LEYF-owned Nurseries. The research was carried out as follows.

- Practitioners who were familiar to the children were used rather than an external person, to avoid some of the difficulties encountered by previously published researchers.

- A pack with guidance notes was employed to ensure that each nursery used the same method of evidence collection:

  - The pack consisted of a frame with Velcro.

  - Names of all staff members in the nursery *except* the member of staff designated to carry out the research.

  - Pictures of activities carried out inside the nursery deliberately did not show any adults in order to avoid any covert suggestions of gender that the children might choose.

It was clearly stated that the interviewer must be a woman. Underneath the names were laminated photos of selected activities. Staff were instructed to use the ones provided, and not to use any others.

The activities agreed were based on the stereotypical assumptions about gender roles from the current research:

- rough-and-tumble play/gymnastics;

- superhero play;

- cooking;

- construction;

- science experiments (minibeast activity involving a member of staff holding the insect);

- dolls (washing);

- stories and songs;

- football;

- trains;

- skipping ropes.

Research methodology

Using all the necessary ethical checks and consents, four children were identified (two boys and two girls) aged three years plus, who had been in the nursery for some time and were familiar with all the activities on the list.

A consistent member of staff was allocated to lead the process and to remain separate from any of the nominated activities in order to limit the chances that the child would feel obliged to pick the member of staff doing the research.

The staff member then conducted a one-to-one activity, lasting no more than five minutes, five times in one week.

Case studies

At the end of the research project LEYF carried out three case studies with:

- David Stevens (LEYF manager);

- Ricky Bullen, (LEYF deputy manager);

- Bryan Mansiamina (apprentice).

The intention was to gauge their reactions to the research findings, and to find out more in order to plan future strategies to encourage more men into the profession. It was important to learn about things they had encountered, especially how people had reacted to their decision to work in early years childcare, and to ask what improvements could be made in terms of recruitment and retention. Some of their comments are included in this chapter to illustrate some of the issues.

Research questions

The following questions were asked:

- What is your name and age?

- How long have you been working in early years childcare?

- Did you do any other job before working in childcare?

- What/who gave you the idea of working in childcare?

- What was the reaction of your friends/family?

- What have been your best personal experiences of the job?

- What have been the bad personal experiences of the job?

- Why do we need more men in childcare?

- How does having a male role model benefit a child's nursery experience (eg dads/ single parents)?

- Have you encountered any difficulties as a male carer with parents/other carers?

- The LEYF survey raised a number of issues regarding male childcarers. Which of those surprised you, if any? Why?

- Has the survey contributed to a change in your practice?

The children's responses

When the children's responses were examined and compared to those from the staff there were some very interesting and sometimes surprising results. It was important to look more closely at those figures to see whether boys were choosing to play with male practitioners and girls with female practitioners. The data showed, however, that 13 per cent of boys and 4.3 per cent of girls chose to play with men, but 17.3 per cent of girls and 8.6 per cent of boys chose to play with women (see Table 7).

Likewise, with rough-and-tumble play, 41 per cent of the staff felt male input was valuable, and 43.4 per cent of children opted for this activity. Surprisingly, of the total number of children only 4.3 per cent were boys and 39.1 per cent were girls (see Table 8).

The remaining 21.7 per cent of boys in the research group chose rough-and-tumble with women.

Of the staff, 50 per cent believed football was an area of play that men could offer the children that they perceived as value-added. Only 43 per cent of children opted to play football – surprisingly perhaps, that was 26 per cent girls and 17.2 per cent boys.

This flies very much in the face of pre-existing research that indicates that men engage children much more than women in rough-and-tumble and physical play. The very low take-up of construction play was unexpected, with 22 per cent of staff flagging its importance but only 4.3 per cent (one girl) choosing to carry out the activity with a woman.

Of the staff, 19.6 per cent believed that superhero play was an activity where men could bring something special. Of the children, 52 per cent opted for this activity: 47.8 per cent boys and 4.3 per cent girls. This was obviously an activity where children preferred to a significant degree to play with men.

Table 7 Percentage of children preferring male/female play

Gender of preferred professional	% male children opting for professional	% female children opting for professional
Male	13	4.3 (1 girl)
Female	8.6	17.3

Table 8 Percentage of children opting for rough-and-tumble play with male professional

Type of play activity with male professional	% male children opting for this activity	% female children opting for this activity
Rough-and-tumble	4.3	39.1

Table 9 Percentage of children opting for superhero play with male professional

Type of play activity with male professional	% male children opting for this activity	% female children opting for this activity
Superhero play	47.8	4.3 (1 girl)

Only 10.7 per cent of staff thought that cooking was an area where men could add to children's experience. However, 43.5 per cent of children opted to cook: 26 per cent of boys and 17.2 per cent of girls. It was fascinating to note that the numbers were identical: ie 13 per cent of boys chose to work with men and 13 per cent of girls chose to work with women, while 8.6 per cent of boys chose to work with women and 8.6 per cent girls chose to work with men.

The doll play was perhaps predictable. Only 1.8 per cent of staff thought this was an important area for men to be role models. All 95.6 per cent of the children, 87 per cent of whom were girls, opted to play with women. However, since 75.0 per cent of staff believed it was very important for men to be seen as nurturing and sensitive role models, and 66.0 per cent felt they could change society's attitudes towards men working with children, perhaps consideration needs to be given as to whether staff too are actually adding to stereotypical images in areas of play that are thought to be 'female'.

The take-up by children for skipping and trains was identical at 17.2 per cent, and in their choice of whether or not to work with a man or woman, 4.3 per cent of girls chose a man, 4.3 per cent of girls chose a woman and 8.6 per cent of boys chose a woman (see Table 10). The staff expectation was 12.5 per cent for trains and 3.6 per cent for skipping. This was perhaps surprising, as trains are often stereotypically seen as something boys prefer, and the adult male role models that one sees skipping are usually sportsmen in training.

In both activities no boys chose a male professional.

Table 10 *Percentage of take up by children of skipping and trains*

Type of play activity with female professional	% male children opting for this activity	% female children opting for this activity
Skipping	8.6	4.3
Trains	8.6	4.3

Table 11 *Percentage of children opting for stories and songs*

Type of play activity with female professional	% male children opting for this activity	% female children opting for this activity
Stories and songs	26	4.3 (1 girl)

Of the staff, 12.5 per cent thought science was an important area of learning for men, but 39.1 per cent of the children chose it, and of those only 8.6 per cent were boys. During the 1970s and 1980s, the consistent underperformance of girls in mathematics and science was a major concern. These issues seem to have been successfully addressed, and GCSE results show year on year that girls are catching up and even overtaking boys in what was once considered to be a 'male' subject.

Key findings

Perhaps one area that needs particular note is that of stories and songs. Only 5.4 per cent of staff felt it was significant for men to bring an additional perspective; 30.4 per cent of children opted for this activity, of which 26 per cent were boys and 4.3 per cent girls (see Table 11). All chose to work with women.

It is interesting to note that there were no recorded comments about gender during the activity research. Staff logged what the children said, and it was all about the activity itself and not about the staff members.

Research summary

In summary, the research was found to be valuable as a means of allowing children's voices to be heard. Children's voices must continue to be heard, as clearly they prove the point that what they want is often different from what adults think they want. It would be helpful to get an even clearer picture by repeating the research using a slightly more refined method, in a way that collects data from a larger number of children over a longer period of time and with a wider range of staff, beginning in London and then beyond.

> *What interested me was that the children really chose because of the staff ability with activities rather than by their gender.*
>
> David Stevens (LEYF manager)

Critical questions

»   *How would you ensure that children's voices are heard?*

»   *How could you include children in action research?*

»   *If you were carrying out the research, would you have asked the same questions? If not, what would you have asked?*

»   *Considering the research findings, in what way does a male role model impact on a child's learning experience?*

»   *How does the male practitioner impact on the children's choice of activities?*

Supporting male staff to build a virtuous cycle of well-being

> *Success will look great when we are noted for our good practice and professional confidence as early years practitioners rather than being noteworthy for being male.*
>   Ricky Bullen (LEYF deputy manager)

The London Early Years Foundation has long been exploring why it is important to encourage men into childcare. It believes that the emphasis on poor pay, lack of promotion opportunities, poor status, fear of accusations of abuse and paedophilia, discomfort working in such a highly female work environment, and an expectation that one man can address the shortfall of positive male roles in so many children's lives detracts from the main question, which is *Do you want to work with children?*

The lack of encouragement and even hostility by others to men joining the early years childcare profession demonstrates the need to focus on work with secondary schools and job centres to raise the awareness of career opportunities in the sector. A high level of male-friendly publicity and advertising is required to raise public awareness and to dispel many existing stereotypes: especially the surprisingly commonplace assumption about the type of men attracted to childcare. This is not helped by negative media campaigns, often based on supposition that infiltrates society and confirms, rather than challenges, negative assumptions.

Internal policy changes are required, such as LEYF's policy to put, whenever possible, two male practitioners together into a nursery to help to alleviate feelings of social isolation and of being *the token male*. There is also an intention to ask male staff members to mentor male students and apprentices, or newly appointed male staff members. A direct response to the research was the launch of a *London Network of Men in Childcare*. This was considered a vehicle to help share good practice, experiences and successes. In the longer term it may provide another means of preventing male practitioners from feeling so isolated. Male practitioners are uniquely placed to dispel images of childcare being a 'female' occupation and nurseries a 'female' preserve. They have opportunities to link more closely with fathers and to help to raise their confidence and parenting skills.

The opportunity for men to lead research about issues that affect them is the most identified purpose of the Network. Members welcomed the chance to create a place where they, along with fellow practitioners, can make sense of what they have learnt, experienced and observed over the years to the benefit of the wider early years community. Practitioners are often so driven by the need to respond to the deluge of day-to-day pressures that they have neither the time nor the inclination to consider more abstract ideas or to reflect upon broader patterns and the wider picture. The members of the Network expressed a willingness to work with universities – a point also perceived by Koshy and Pascal (2011, p 438), who observed a growing popularity among practitioners for undertaking research with researchers in universities. Many participants saw this as an opportunity to develop their leadership, not just personally but as leaders of men in childcare: a prerequisite for excellence.

> We are pioneers in breaking down prejudice and now we are getting men of all ages and backgrounds becoming the first established generation of men in childcare. For example our Men in Childcare Network is a really mixed group.
>
> Bryan Mansiamina (LEYF apprentice)

The staff perception that men don't add any value to reading stories and singing, also confirmed by the majority of children, who chose female staff for these activities, needs to be addressed. Challenging this view is critical, given the worrying data about boys' literacy skills and the continuing negative attitude that reading is for girls. This will be particularly useful with regard to the findings of research into language and literacy carried out with small boys. This was summed up by the National Literacy Trust (National Literacy Trust, 2012), which found that only one in four boys read outside class every day, meaning that:

> By the time they reach school, many boys are already lagging behind in literacy: at age five, there is a gap of 11 percentage points between boys' and girls' achievement in reading.

Unless men provide positive gender modelling in literacy, boys attending nursery – particularly those who do not have male reading role models at home – will continue to see reading and literacy as something that is 'done by girls and women'. Attention to the role of men in supporting children's literacy, particularly that of boys, presents exciting opportunities to devise ways of working with fathers to raise awareness of the importance of reading with their sons and being seen reading for pleasure. As any future success in education is predicated on competent literacy, then failing to address this almost confirms failure for many male children.

Critical questions

» *How would you encourage more involvement by fathers?*

» *Do you think that by having male practitioners you would be able to engage better with fathers?*

» *Would having male practitioners create better opportunities for improving boys' literacy outcomes?*

» *What would you do if parents objected to having a male practitioner?*

Critical reflections

This chapter has discussed the importance of having both men and women in caring roles.

» *There is a need to eliminate negative images of sexual stereotyping and assumptions about male and female roles which has made it difficult to recruit men into careers in working with young children.*

» *The emphases on poor pay, lack of promotion opportunities, poor status, fear of accusations of abuse and paedophilia and discomfort working in such a highly female work environment mask the actual reasons for few men in childcare and therefore make it difficult to respond effectively to these.*

» *Secondary schools and job centres need to raise the awareness of career opportunities in the sector. More publicity and advertising designed to attract men of different ages is required to promote childcare as needing to be a gender-balanced profession.*

» *Many children, especially pre-secondary school, lack a male role model in their life, so both boys and girls can benefit from contact with positive male role models in early years and primary school contexts.*

» *The LEYF research has demonstrated that male practitioners have helped to build closer involvement by fathers. A male presence on the staff showed fathers that men are welcome in the early childhood setting and that men can play a part in children's care and education, encouraging fathers to become more involved.*

» *There is a belief that men bring a more active and physical approach to the way they interact with their own children and with children in general. But the LEYF research showed the opposite: children chose female as well as male practitioners for rough-and-tumble play. However, the boys saw reading and literacy activities as female and the organisation needed to consider ways to address this, particularly in the light of young boys' lower literacy levels.*

» *Male practitioners are uniquely placed to dispel images of childcare being a 'female' occupation and nurseries being a 'female preserve'. They have opportunities to link more closely with fathers and to help raise their confidence and parenting skills. Most importantly there is a need for all practitioners to understand that male childcare adds strength to the well-being cycle for children.*

Further reading

Potter, C., Olley, R. (2012) *Engaging Fathers in the Early Years: A Practitioner's Guide*. London: Continuum.

This reflective but practical guide draws on the expertise of a range of professionals in discussing the engagement of fathers in their children's early development. It examines current policy frameworks and provides practitioners with strategies and evaluation techniques for recruiting, engaging and retaining the involvement of fathers.

Tett, L.; Riddell, S. (2006) *Gender and Teaching: Where Have All the Men Gone?* Edinburgh: Dunedin Academic Press.

An in-depth analysis of the reasons why men are less likely to choose to become teachers based on research into the gender balance of teaching in Scotland. The issues dealt with and the lessons to be learnt from this study are of wider significance to early years practitioners.

Browne, N. (2004) *Gender Equity in the Early Years*. Maidenhead: Open University Press.

This book provides a critical evaluation of the extent to which current early years policies and practice promote gender equity, in particular the rationale for the drive to employ more men in the early years field.

References

Abel, E.L; Sokol, R.J. (1987) Incidence of Fetal Alcohol Syndrome and Economic Impact of FAS-related Anomalies: Drug Alcohol Syndrome and Economic Impact of FAS-related Anomalies. *Drug and Alcohol Dependency*, 19(1): 51–70.

Adoption Act (1976) London: HMSO.

Aeltermann, A.; Engels, N.; Van Petegem, K.; Verheghe, J.P. (2007) The Well-being of Teachers in Flanders. *Educational Studies*, 33(3): 285–97.

Afasic UK (2004) *Selective Mutism*. Available from www.afasiccymru.org.uk/glossary/glossary%2006.pdf. Accessed 24 April 2012.

Ainsworth, M.D.S.; Blehar, M.; Waters, E.; Wall, S. (1978) *Patterns of Attachment*. Hillsdale, NJ: Erlbaum.

Aldgate, J. (2007) The Place of Attachment Theory in Social Work with Children and Families, in Lishman, J. (ed) *Handbook for Practice Learning in Social Work and Social Care*. London: Jessica Kingsley.

Aldgate, J.; Jeffrey, C.; Jones, D.; Rose, W. (2006) *The Developing World of the Child*. London: Jessica Kingsley.

Allan, G. (2010) Substance Use: What Are the Risks?, in Hothersall, S.J; Maas-Lowit, M. (eds) *Need, Risk and Protection in Social Work Practice*. Exeter: Learning Matters.

Allan, J. (1993) Male Elementary Teachers: Experiences and Perspectives, in Williams, C.L. (ed) *Doing 'Women's Work': Men in Non-Traditional Occupations*. Newbury Park, CA: Sage.

Anderson, L.M.; Anderson, J. (2010) Barney and Breakfast: Messages about Food and Eating in Pre-school Television Shows and How They May Impact the Development of Eating Behaviours in Children. *Early Child Development and Care*, 180(10): 1323–36.

Anning, A. and Hall, D. in Anning, A. and Ball, M. (2008) *Improving Services for Young Children: From Sure Start to Children's Centres*. London: Sage.

Anon. (2012) 'Berated, Frozen Out, Colluded Against ...': Why One Male Practitioner Knows He Is Definitely Not Welcome. *Nursery World*, 2 October. Available from www.nurseryworld.co.uk/article/1152918/berated-frozen-out-colluded-against-why-one-male-practitioner-knows-definitely-not-welcome. Accessed 13 July 2013.

Arrow, P.; Raheb, J.; Miller, M. (2013) *BMC Public Health*, 13(1): 1–9.

Arthur, L. (1993) *Programming and Planning in Early Childhood Settings*. San Diego: Harcourt Brace Jovanovich.

Australia Bureau of Statistics (2008) *The People of Australia: Statistics from the 2006 Census*. Canberra: Department of Immigration and Citizenship.

BBC (2011) *Weaning before Six Months May Help Breastfed Babies*. Available at www.bbc.co.uk/news/health-12180052. Accessed 1 April 2013.

BBC (2013) *Childcare Ratios: 'We will find way forward', Says Cameron*, www.bbc.co.uk/news/uk-politics-22564178. Accessed 18 May 2013.

Blatchford, P.; Battle, S.; Mays, J. (1982) *The First Transition: Home to Pre-school. A Report on the 'Transition from Home to Pre-school' Project*. Windsor: NFER–Nelson.

Bligh, C. (2011) The Silent Experiences of Young Bilingual Learners: A Small Scale Sociocultural Exploration. PhD thesis, The Open University.

Blount, J.M. (2005) *Fit to Teach: Same-Sex Desire, Gender, and School Work in the Twentieth Century*. Albany: State University of New York Press.

Bowlby, J. (1953) *Child Care and the Growth of Love*. Harmondsworth: Penguin.

Bowlby, J. (1958) The Nature of a Child's Tie to His Mother. *The International Journal of Psycho-analysis*, 39: 350–53.

Braun, V.; Clarke, V. (2006) Using Thematic Analysis in Psychology. *Qualitative Research in Psychology*, 3: 77–101.

Briner, R.; Dewberry, C. (2007) *Staff Well-being Is Key to School Success: A Research Study into the Links between Staff Well-being and School Performance*. London: Department of Organizational Psychology, Birkbeck, University of London, in partnership with Worklife Support.

Bronfenbrenner, U. (1979) *The Ecology of Human Development: Experiments by Nature and Design*. Cambridge, MA: Harvard University Press.

Brown, P. 'Naming and framing: the social construction of diagnosis and illness' in *Journal of Health and Social Behavior* (1995): 34–52.

Browne, N. (2004) *Gender Equity in the Early Years*. Maidenhead: Open University Press.

Bruner, J. (1996) *The Culture of Education*. Cambridge, MA: Harvard University Press.

Cameron, C. (2001) Promise or Problem? A Review of the Literature on Men Working in Early Childhood Services. *Gender, Work and Organization*, 8(4): 430–53.

Cameron, C. (2007) Men in the Nursery Revisited: Issues of Male Workers and Professionalism. *Contemporary Issues in Early Childhood*, 7(1): 68–79.

Cameron, C.; Moss, P. (1999) Men as Carers for Young Children: An Introduction, in Owen, C.; Cameron, C.; Moss, P. (eds) *Men as Workers in Services for Young Children: Issues of a Mixed Gender Workforce*. London: Institute of Education, University of London.

Cameron, C.; Moss, P. (2004) *Gender Issues in Care Work in Europe, Thomas Coram Research Unit*. London: Institute of Education, University of London.

Cavendish, L. (2011) Does Day Care Damage Your Baby? One Mother's View ... *The Telegraph*, 13 September. Available at www.telegraph.co.uk/women/mother-tongue/8758117/Does-day-care-damage-your-baby-One-mothers-view.html. Accessed 19 July 2013.

Channel 4 (2013) *Childcare Reforms Plans in 'Chaos', Labour Says*, www.channel4.com/news/childcare-ratios-reform-nick-clegg-government-plans. Accessed 10 May 2013.

Children Act (1989) London: HMSO.

Children Act (2002) London: The Stationery Office.

Children Act (2004) London: The Stationery Office.

Children's Society (2012a) *Promoting Positive Well-being for Children*. Available from www.childrenssociety.org.uk/sites/default/files/tcs/promoting_positive_well-being_for_children_final.pdf. Accessed 12 March 2013.

Children's Society (2012b) *The Good Childhood Report*. Available from www.childrenssociety.org.uk/sites/default/files/tcs/good_childhood_report_2012_final_0.pdf. Accessed 1 January 2013.

Chodorow, N. (1978) *The Reproduction of Mothering: Psychoanalysis and the Sociology of Gender*. Berkeley: University of California Press.

Clark, A. (2000) *Listening to Young Children: Perspectives, Possibilities and Problems*. Paper presented to the 10th European Conference on Quality in Early Childhood Education, EECERA Conference, London, 29 August–1 September.

Clark, A.; Moss, P. (2001) *Listening to Young Children: The Mosaic Approach*. London: National Children's Bureau.

Clark, A.; Moss, P.; Kjorholt, A.T. (2005) *Beyond Listening: Children's Perspectives on Early Childhood Services*. Bristol: Policy Press.

Clarke, P. (1996) Investigating Second Language Acquisition in Preschools. PhD thesis, Latrobe University. Published in Clarke (2009).

Clarke, P. (2009) *Supporting Children Learning English as a Second Language in the Early Years (Birth to Six Years)*. Melbourne: Victorian Curriculum and Assessment Authority.

Cline, T. and Baldwin, S. (2004) *Selective mutism in children*, 2nd ed. London: Whurr Publishers.

Cohen, J.; Kay, J. (1994) *Taking Drugs Seriously: A Parent's Guide to Young People's Drug Use*. London: Thorsons.

Community Care Inspiring Excellence in Social Care (2013) *Multi-agency Safeguarding Centre for Children's Referrals*, www.communitycare.co.uk/articles/07/06/2011/116936/multi-agency-safeguarding-centre-for-childrens-referrals.htm. Accessed 5 May 2013.

Conteh, J. (2003) *Succeeding in Diversity: Culture, Language and Learning in Primary Classrooms*. London: Trentham.

Conti, G.; Heckman, J.J. (2012) *The Economics of Child Well-being*. Cambridge, MA: National Bureau of Economic Research.

Cottrell, S. (2005) *Critical thinking skills*. Palgrave Macmillan

Croghan, L.; Craven, R. (1982) Elective Mutism: Learning from the Analysis of a Successful Case History. *Paediatric Psychology*, 7(1): 85–93.

Currer, C. (2001) *Responding to Grief: Dying, Bereavement and Social Care*. Basingstoke: Palgrave.

Dahlberg, G.; Moss, P.; Pence, A. (1999) *Beyond Quality in Early Childhood Education: Postmodern Perspectives*. London: Falmer Press.

Daniel, B. (2006) Early Childhood: Zero to Four Years, in Aldgate, J.; Jones, D.; Rose, W.; Jeffrey, C. (eds) *The Developing World of the Child*. London. Jessica Kingsley.

Daniel, P.; Ivatts, J. (1998) *Children and Social Policy*. Basingstoke: Macmillan.

Darder, A. (ed) (2002) *Reinventing Paulo Friere: A Pedagogy of Love*. Boulder, CO: Westview Press.

Davis-Kean, P.E.; Sandler, H.M. (2001) A Meta-analysis of Measures of Self-esteem for Young Children: A Framework for Future Measures. *Child Development*, 72(3): 887–906.

Daycare Trust (2011) *Finding and Choosing Childcare*, www.daycaretrust.org.uk/pages/quick-guide-to-childcare-finding-and-choosing-childcare-431.html. Accessed 4 April 2013.

DCSF (Department for Children, Schools and Families) (2007) *Early Years Foundation Stage*. Nottingham: DCSF Publications.

DCSF (Department for Children, Schools and Families) (2008) *Every Child a Talker: Guidance for Early Language Lead Practitioners. Third Instalment*. Available from http://earlylearningconsultancy.co.uk/wp-content/uploads/2010/12/ECAT-Third-Instalment.pdf. Accessed 20 October 2012.

de Braal, B. (2009) Depression in Childhood: Is There an Epidemic? *School Health Journal*, 5(2): 18–20.

Delgado Gaitan, C. (2006) *Building Culturally Responsive Classrooms: A Guide for K-6 Teachers*. Thousand Oaks, CA: Corwin Press.

Demuynck, K.; Peeters, J. (2006) *Ouderparticipatie, ook voor vaders*. Gent: VBJK.

DfE (Department for Education) (2012a) *Primary National Curriculum (Draft)*. Available from www.education.gov.uk/schools/teachingandlearning/curriculum/primary?page=1. Accessed 15 December 2012.

DfE (Department for Education) (2012b) *Statutory Framework for the Early Years Foundation Stage*. DFE-00023-2012. Available from www.education.gov.uk/publications/standard/AllPublications/Page1/. Accessed 10 October 2012.

DfE (Department for Education) (2013a) *Managing Medicines in Schools*, www.education.gov.uk/schools/pupilsupport/pastoralcare/b0013771/managing-medicines. Accessed 20 July 2013.

DfE (Department for Education) (2013b) *Working Together to Safeguard Children*. Available from www.education.gov.uk/aboutdfe/statutory/g00213160/working-together-to-safeguard-children. Accessed 21 July 2013.

DFE/DH (2011) Supporting Families in the Foundation Years, Department of Health and Department of Education, UK Government.

DfES (Department for Education and Skills); DH (Department of Health) (2005) *Managing Medicines in Schools and Early Years Settings*. London: DfES. Available from www.education.gov.uk/publications/standard/publicationDetail/Page1/DFES-1448–2005.

DH (Department of Health) (1996) *Focus on Teenagers: Research into Practice*. London: HMSO.

DH (Department of Health) (2004) *National Service Framework for Children, Young People andMaternity Services*. Available online from http://webarchive.nationalarchives.gov.uk/20130401151715/www.education.gov.uk/publications/eOrderingDownload/DH-40496PDF.pdf. Accessed 20 July 2013.

DH (Department of Health) (2007) Making it better for children and young people.

Di Gioacchino, D. (2012) 'Parental Care, Children's Cognitive Abilities and Economic Growth: The Role of Fathers' in *Theoretical Economics* 2.

Drury, R. (2007) *Young Bilingual Learners at Home and School: Researching Multilingual Voices*. Stoke-on-Trent: Trentham.

Edwards, A. (2012) It's a Manny's World! Teenager Becomes First Male Undergraduate at Prestigious 'Mary Poppins' Nanny College. *Mail Online*, 6 September. Available from www.dailymail.co.uk/news/article-2199043/Its-mannys-world-Teenager-male-undergraduate-prestigious-Mary-Poppins-nanny-college.html. Accessed 22 July 2013.

Edwards, G. (2005) *Matters of Substance: Is Legislation the Right Answer – or the Wrong Question?* London: Penguin.

Engel, G.L. (1980) 'The clinical application of the biopsychosocial model' in *Am J Psychiatry* 137(5): 535–544.

European Commission (2011) *Early Childhood Education and Care: Providing All Our Children with the Best Start for the World of Tomorrow*. Brussels.

European Commission Network on Childcare (1996) *Quality Targets in Services for Young Children and Other Measures to Reconcile the Employment and Family Responsibilities of Men and Women, Paper 3*. Brussels.

European Parliament Committee on Women's Rights and Gender Equality (2012) *Draft Report on Eliminating Gender Stereotypes in the EU* (2012/2116 (INI)).

Fagan, J. (1996) Principles for Developing Male Involvement Programs in Early Childhood Settings: A Personal Experience. *Young Children*, 51(4): 64–71.

Fahlberg, V. (1994) *A Child's Journey through Placement*. London: British Agencies for Adoption and Fostering.

Farquhar, S.-E. (2012) *Recruitment and Employment of Men in Early Childhood Teaching, Childcare, Kindergarten and Home-based Early Childhood Education*. Porirua, NZ: Child Forum Research Network.

Farquhar, S.-E.; Cablk, L.; Buckingham, A.; Butler, D.; Ballantyne, R. (2006) *Men at Work: Sexism in Early Childhood Education*. Porirua, NZ: Child Forum Research Network.

FASD Trust (2013) *The FASD Trust*, www.fasdtrust.co.uk. Accessed 21 July 2013.

Fattore, T.; Mason, J.; Watson, E. (2007) Children's Conceptualisations of Their Well-being. *Social Indicators Research*, 80(1): 5–29.

Fattore, T.; Mason, J.; Watson, E. (2009) When Children Are Asked about Their Well-being: Towards a Framework for Guiding Policy. *Child Indicators Research*, 21(1): 57–77.

Festinger, L. (1957) *A Theory of Cognitive Dissonance*. Stanford, CA: Stanford University Press.

Fewtrell, M.; Wilson, D.C.; Booth, I.; Lucas, A. (2011) Six Months of Exclusive Breast Feeding: How Good Is the Evidence? *BMJ*, 342: c5955.

Fifield, S.; Swain, H.L. (2002) Heteronormativity and Common Sense in Science (Teacher) Education, in Kisson, R.M. (ed) *Getting Ready for Benjamin: Preparing Teachers for Sexual Diversity in the Classroom*. Lanham, MD: Rowman and Littlefield.

Fisher, A. (2001) *Critical Thinking, an introduction*. Cambridge University Press

Fleer, M.; Anning, A.; Cullen, J. (2004) A Framework for Conceptualising Early Education, in Anning, A.; Cullen, J.; Fleer, M. (eds) *Early Childhood Education: Society and Culture*. London: Sage.

Flewitt, R. (2005) Is Every Child's Voice Heard? Researching the Different Ways 3-year-old Children Communicate and Make Meaning at Home and in a Preschool Playgroup. *Early Years: An International Journal of Research and Development*, 25(3): 207–22.

Fox Harding, L. (1997) *Perspectives on Child Care Policy*. 2nd edn. London: Longman.

Gee, J.; Green, J. (1998) Discourse Analysis, Learning and Social Practice: A Methodological Study. *Review of Research in Education*, 23: 119–69.

Gentleman, A. (2010) The Great Nursery Debate. *Guardian*, 2 October. Available at www.guardian.co.uk/lifeandstyle/2010/oct/02/nurseries-childcare-pre-school-cortisol. Accessed 14 June 2013.

Gerhardt, S. (2006) 'Why love matters: How affection shapes a baby's brain' *Infant Observation* 9(3): 305–309.

Gopnik, A.; Meltzoff, A.; Kuhl, P. (1999) *How Babies Think: The Science of Childhood*. London: Weidenfeld and Nicolson.

Gosse, D.; Facchinetti, A. (2012) What's in a Male? *Education Today*, 12(4): 26–40.

GOV.UK (2013) *Simplifying the Welfare System and Making Sure Work Pays*, www.dwp.gov.uk/policy/disability/personal-independence-payment/. Accessed 21 July 2013.

Greenberg, J.P. (2011) The Impact of Maternal Education on Children's Enrollment in Early Childhood Education and Care. *Children and Youth Services Review*, 33(7): 1049–57.

Greene, S.; Hill, M. (2005) Researching Children's Experiences: Methods and Methodological Issues. Cited in Greene, S.; Hogan, D. (eds) *Researching Children's Experience: Approaches and Methods*. London: Sage.

Greenfield, S. (2000) *The Private Life of the Brain*. London: Penguin.

Greenfield, S. (2011) Nursery Home Visits: Rhetoric and Realities. *Journal of Early Childhood Research*. doi: 10.1177/1476718X11407983.

Haase, M. (2008) I Don't Do the Mothering Role that Lots of Female Teachers Do: Male Teachers, Gender, Power and Social Organisation. *British Journal of Sociology of Education*, 29(6): 597–608.

Hall, D. and Elliman, D. (2004) *Health for All Children*. Oxford University Press

Halpern, D.F. (1996) *Thought and Knowledge: an introduction to critical thinking*. Mahwah: Lawrence Erlbaum

Hammond, M. and Collins, R. (1991) *Self-Directed Learning: Critical Practice*. ERIC.

Hancock, R.; Gillen, J. (2007) Safe Places in Domestic Spaces: Two-year-olds at Play in Their Homes. *Children's Geographies*, 5(4): 337–51.

Hand, A.; McDonnell, E.; Honarl, B.; Sharry, J. (2013) A Community Led Approach to Delivery of the Parents Plus Children's Programme for the Parents of Children Aged 6–11. *International Journal of Clinical Health and Psychology*, 13(2): 81–90.

Hardman, C. (1973) Can There Be an Anthropology of Children? *Journal of the Anthropology Society of Oxford*, 4(1): 85–99.

Harrison, L.J.; Ungerer, J.A. (2002) Maternal Employment and Infant–Mother Attachment Security at 12 Months Postpartum. *Developmental Psychology*, 38(5): 758–73.

HCPC (Health and Care Professions Council) (2013) *HCPC*, www.hcpc-uk.org. Accessed 21 July 2013.

HEMAS (Hampshire Ethnic Minority Achievement Service) (2003) *Selective Mutism: Selective Mutism or the 'Silent Period'?* Available from www3.hants.gov.uk/education/ema/ema.../ema-mutism.htm. Accessed 12 October 2012.

Hooyman, N.; Kramer, B. (2006) *Living through Loss: Interventions across the Lifespan*. New York: Columbia University Press.

Howe, D. (1995) *Attachment Theory for Social Work Practice*. Basingstoke: Macmillan.

Howe, D. (2001) Attachment, in Howarth, J. (ed) *The Child's World: Assessing Children in Need*. London: Jessica Kingsley.

Hughes, J. (2012) Social Work with Children with Disabilities and Their Familes, in O'Loughlin, M.; O'Loughlin, S. (eds) *Social Work with Children and Families*. 3rd edn. Exeter: Learning Matters.

IPSOS Mori (2003) *Men and Childcare UK* (poll).

IPSOS Mori Social Research Institute; Nairn, A. (2011) *Children's Well-being in UK, Sweden and Spain: The Role of Inequality and Materialism. A Qualitative Study.*

Janis, I.L., and Mann, L. (1977) *Decision making: A psychological analysis of conflict, choice, and commitment.* Free Press.

Jensen, J. (1996) *Men as Workers in Childcare Services.* Brussels: European Commission Network on Childcare.

Jensen, J. (1998) Men as Workers in Childcare Services, in Owen, C.; Cameron, C.; Moss, P. (eds) *Men as Workers in Services for Young Children: Issues of Gender Workforce.* London: Institute of Education.

Jewett, C. (1984) *Helping Children Cope with Separation and Loss.* London: Batsford.

Johnson, S.P. (2008) *The Status of Male Teachers in Public Education Today.* Education Policy Brief 6(4). Bloomington: Centre for Evaluation and Education Policy (CEEP), Indiana University.

Kagan, S. (1989) 'The structural approach to cooperative learning' in *Educational Leadership* 47(4): 12–15.

Kakuma, R. (2002) *The Optimal Duration of Exclusive Breastfeeding: A Systematic Review.* Geneva: World Health Organization.

Kalliopuska, M. (1994) Relations of Retired People and Their Grandchildren. *Psychological Reports*, 75: 1083–88. Cited in Meyers and Swiebert (1999).

Kato, K. (2001) Exploring 'Cultures of Learning': A Case of Japanese and Australian Classrooms. *Journal of Intercultural Studies*, 22(1): 51–67.

Kato, K. (2010) Silence as Participation: The Case of Japanese Students. *Journal of Multiculturalism in Education*, 6(2): 13.

Kellet, M. (2010) *Rethinking Children and Research.* London: Continuum.

Kemshall, H.; Pritchard, J. (eds) (2002) *Good Practice in Risk Assessment and Risk Management.* London: Jessica Kingsley.

King, J.R. (1998) *Uncommon Caring: Learning from Men who Teach Young Children.* New York: Teachers College Press.

King, A. (1995) 'Designing the instructional process to enhance critical thinking across the curriculum' in *Teaching of Psychology* 22(1): 13–17.

Kolucki, B.; Lemish, D. (2011) *Communicating with Children: Principles and Practices to Nurture, Inspire, Excite, Educate and Heal.* New York: UNICEF.

Koshy, V.; Pascal, C. (2011) Nurturing the Young Shoots of Talent: Using Action Research for Exploration and Theory Building. *European Early Childhood Education Research Journal*, 19(4): 433–50.

Kuhn, M.; Eischen, W. (1997) *Leveraging the Aptitude and Ability of Eight Year-Old Adults ... and Other Wonders of Technology: How to Be Number One in the Youth Market.* ESOMAR conference. Copenhagen.

Laevers, F.; Heylen, L. (eds) (2003) Involvement of Children and Teacher Style: Insights from an International Study on Experiential Learning. Studia Paedagogica, 35. Leuven: Leuven University Press.

Lamb, M. (2000) *The Role of the Father in Child Development.* New York: John Wiley.

Lancaster, L.; Broadbent, V. (2003) *Listening to Young Children.* Maidenhead: Open University Press.

Lave, J.; Wenger, E. (1991) *Situated Learning: Legitimate Peripheral Participation.* Cambridge: Cambridge University Press.

Layard, R.; Dunn, J. (2009) *A Good Childhood: Searching for Values in a Competitive Age.* London: Penguin.

Li, J.; Johnson, S.E.; Han, W.J.; Andrews, S.; Kendall, G.; Strazdins, L.; Dockery, A.M. (2012) *Parents' Nonstandard Work and Child Well-being: A Critical Review of the Existing Literature.* CLMR Discussion Paper Series. Available from www.pandora.nla.gov.au/pan/102621/20120831-0000/1202.pdf. Accessed 13 July 2013.

Local Authority and Social Services Act (1970) London: HMSO.

Maas-Lowit, M. (2010) Capacity and Incapacity, in Hothersall, S.J.; Maas-Lowit, M. (eds) *Need, Risk and Protection in Social Work Practice.* Exeter: Learning Matters.

McConkey, R.; Bhurgri, S. (2003) Children with Autism Attending Preschool Facilities: The Experiences and Perceptions of Staff. *Early Child Development and Care*, 173: 443–52.

McLeod, A. (2008) Listening to Children: A Practitioner's Guide. London: Jessica Kingsley.

Magraw, I.; Dimmock, E. (2006) *Silence and Presence: How Adult Attitude Affects the Creativity of Children.* National Teacher Research Panel summary. Available from www.standards.dfes.gov.uk/ntrp/publications/. Accessed 23 August 2008.

Major Provider Group (2011) *Men in Childcare Report.* London.

Matrimonial Causes Act (1973) London: HMSO.

Mayall, B. (2004) Sociologies of Childhood, in Holborn, M. (ed) *Developments in Sociology: An Annual Review.* Ormskirk: Causeway Press.

Mehrotra, S.; Khunyakari, R.; Chunawala, S.; Natarajan, C. (2009) *Evidences of Learning through Collaboration in Design and Technology Tasks in Indian Classrooms*. Mumbai: Homi Bhabha Centre for Science Education, TIFR. Available from http://web.gnowledge.org/episteme3/pro_pdfs/14-swati-rk-sc-cn.pdf. Accessed 12 November 2009.

Meltzoff, A.; Prinz, W. (eds) (2002) *The Imitative Mind: Development, Evolution and Brain Bases*. Cambridge: Cambridge University Press.

Meyers, J.; Swiebert, V. (1999) Grandparents and Step Grandparents: Challenges in Counselling the Extended Blended Family. *Adultspan Journal*, 1(1): 50–60.

Milkie, M.A.; Kendig, S.M.; Nomaguchi, K.M.; Denny, K.E. (2010) Time with Children, Children's Well-being, and Work–Family Balance among Employed Parents. *Journal of Marriage and Family*, 72(5): 1329–43.

Milteer, R.M.; Ginsberg, K.R.; Mulligan, D.A. (2011) *The Importance of Play in Promoting Healthy Child Development and Maintaining Strong Parent–Child Bond: Focus on Children in Poverty*. Available from www.ecementor.org/articles-on-teaching/The_Importance_of_Play_in_Promoting_%20Healthy_Child_Development.pdf. Accessed 20 July 2013.

Ministry of Social Affairs and Health (2006) *Men and Gender Equality: Towards Progressive Policies*. Conference report. Helsinki.

Misuse of Drugs Act (1971) London: HMSO.

Moll, L.; Amanti, C.; Neff, D.; Gonzalez, N. (1992) Funds of Knowledge for Teaching: Using a Qualitative Approach to Connect Homes and Classrooms. *Theory into Practice*, 31(2): 132–41.

Moll, L.; Amanti, C.; Neff, D.; Gonzalez, N. (2005) Funds of Knowledge for Teaching: Using a Qualitative Approach to Connect Homes and Classrooms, in Gonzalez, N.; Moll, L.; Amanti, C. (eds) *Funds of Knowledge: Theorizing Practices in Households, Communities and Classrooms*. London: Lawrence Erlbaum Associates.

Morton, K. (2011) Parents Want Men in Nurseries but Male School Leavers 'Not Interested' in Childcare. *Nursery World*, 26 July. Available from www.nurseryworld.co.uk/article/1081860/parents-want-men-nurseries-male-school-leavers-not-interested-childcare. Accessed 13 July 2013.

Murray, S.B. (1996) We All Love Charles: Men in Childcare and the Social Construction of Gender. *Gender and Society* 10(4): 368–85.

National Literacy Trust (2012) *Boys' Reading Commission: The Report of the All-Party Parliamentary Literacy Group Commission*. London.

Netmums (2013) *How the Modern Family Looks Today*, www.netmums.com/home/netmums-campaigns/how-the-modern-family-looks-today. Accessed 15 May 2013.

NICE (National Institute for Health and Clinical Excellence) (2012) *Social and Emotional Well-being: Early Years*. NICE Public Health Guidance, 40. Available from www.nice.org.uk/nicemedia/live/13941/61149/61149.pdf. Accessed 23 November 2012.

Nutbrown, C. (1982). *Shaking the Foundations of Quality? Why 'Childcare' Policy Must Not Lead to Poor-Quality Early Education and Care*. Available from www.shef.ac.uk/polopoly_fs/1.263201!/file/Shakingthefoundationsofquality.pdf. Accessed 14 July 2013.

Nutbrown, C. (2012) *Foundations for Quality: The Independent Review of Early Education and Childcare Qualifications. Final Report*. London.

Nutbrown, C.; Clough, P. (2006) *Inclusion in the Early Years*. London: Sage.

Oberhuemer, P.; Schreyer, I.; Neuman, M.J. (2010) *Professionals in Early Childhood Education and Care Systems: European Profiles and Perspectives*. Opladen and Farmington Hills, MI: Barbara Budrich.

OECD (Organisation for Economic Co-operation and Development) (2006) *Meeting of the OECD Council at Ministerial Level Paris*, 23–24 May.

OECD (Organisation for Economic Co-operation and Development) (2012) *Meeting of the OECD Council at Ministerial Level Paris*, 23–24 May.

Ofsted (2013) *Early Years and Childcare: For Parents and Carers*, www.ofsted.gov.uk/early-years-and-childcare/for-parents-and-carers/choosing-childcare-provider. Accessed 2 April 2013.

O'Loughlin, M.; O'Loughlin, S. (eds) (2012) *Social Work with Children and Families*. 3rd edn. Exeter: Learning Matters.

ONS (Office for National Statistics) (2013) *Census 2011*, www.ons.gov.uk/census. Accessed 21 July 2013.

Owen, C. (2003) *Men's Work? Changing the Gender Mix of the Childcare and Early Years Workforce*. Facing the Future: Policy Paper no. 6. London: Daycare Trust.

Parke, R. (1996) *Fatherhood: Myths and Realities*. Cambridge, MA: Harvard University Press.

Parke, T.; Drury, R. (2001) Language Development at Home and School: Gains and Losses in Young Bilinguals. *Early Years: An International Journal of Research and Development*, 21(2): 117–27.

Paul, R. and Elder, L. *The Foundation for Critical Thinking* www.criticalthinking.org (accessed 16 September 2013)

Payne, S.; Horn, S.; Relf, M. (1999) *Loss and Bereavement*. Maidenhead: Open University Press.

Peeters, J. (2005) Promoting Diversity and Equality in Early Childhood Care and Education: Men in Childcare, in Schonfeld, H.; O'Brien, S.; Walsh, T. (eds) *Questions of Quality: Proceedings of a Conference on Defining, Assessing and Supporting Quality in Early Childhood Care and Education*. Dublin: CECDE.

Peeters, J. (2007) Including Men in Early Childhood Education: Insights from the European Experience. *Research in Early Childhood Education*, 10: [n.p.].

PHE (Public Health England) (2013a) *HPA: Health Protection Agency Homepage. Protecting People, Preventing Harm, Preparing for Threats*, www.hpa.org.uk. Accessed 21 July 2013.

PHE (Public Health England) (2013b) *Vaccination Schedule*, available from www.hpa.org.uk/web/HPAweb&Page&HPAwebAutoListDate/Page/1204031508623. Accessed 20 July 2013.

Piaget, J. (1955) *The Child's Construction of Reality*. London: Routledge.

Piburn, D. (2006) Gender Equality for a New Generation: Expect Male Involvement in ECE. *Exchange*, 168: 18–22.

Pollard, E.L. and Lee, P.D. (2003) 'Child well-being: a systematic review of the literature' in *Social Indicators Research* 61(1): 59–78.

Potter, C.; Olley, R. (2012) *Engaging Fathers in the Early Years: A Practitioner's Guide*. London: Continuum.

Redcar and Cleveland Children and Young People's Trust (2013) *Child Well-being Operational Guidance Including Common Assessment Framework*, www.redcarclevelandcyptrust.org.uk/ctrust.nsf/WebFullList/07EC073A86DDC2848025748F0049F16D?OpenDocument. Accessed 19 June 2013.

Rinaldi, C. (2005) *In Dialogue with Reggio Emilia*. London: Routledge.

Rogoff, B. (1990) *Apprenticeship in Thinking: Cognitive Development in Social Context*. Oxford: Oxford University Press.

Rogoff, B. (2003) *The Cultural Nature of Human Development*. New York: Oxford University Press.

Rothenberg, P.S. (ed) (2001) *Race, Class and Gender in the United States*, 5th edn. New York: Worth.

Rutter, M. (1985) Resilience in the Face of Adversity: Protective Factors and Resistance to Psychiatric Disorder. *British Journal of Psychiatry*, 147: 598–611.

Ruxton, S. (1992) *'What's He Doing at The Family Centre?' The Dilemmas of Men who Care for Children*. London: National Children's Home.

Sage, R.; Sluckin, A. (2004) *Silent Children: Approaches to Selective Mutism*. Leicester: Smira Publications in Association with the University of Leceister.

Sanders, G.F.; Trygstad, D.W. (1989) Step Grandparents and Grandparents: The View from Young Adults. *Family Relations*, 38: 71–75.

Sanders, J.; Jackson Barnette, J. (eds) (2003) *The Mainstreaming of Evaluation: New Directions for Evaluation*, special issue, 99.

Saville-Troike, M. (1988) Private Speech: Evidence for Second Language Learning Strategies during the 'Silent Period'. *Journal of Child Language*, 15: 567–90.

Sayeed, Z.; Guerin, E. (2000) *Early Years Play: A Happy Medium for Assessment and Intervention*. London: David Fulton.

Schön, D.A. (1983) *The Reflective Practitioner: How Professionals Think in Action*. New York: Basic Books.

Schön, D.A. (1987) *Educating the Reflective Professional*. San Francisco: Jossey-Bass.

Schott, J.; Henley, A. (1996) *Culture, Religion and Childbearing in a Multiracial Society: A Handbook for Health Professionals*. Edinburgh: Butterworth–Heinemann.

Segura-Mora, A. (2002) Friere and the Education of Young Children, in Darder, A. (ed) *Reinventing Paulo Friere: A Pedagogy of Love*. Boulder, CO: Westview Press.

Seifert, K. (1988) The Culture of Early Education and the Preparation of Male Teachers. *Early Child Development and Care*, 38: 69–80.

Shaw, C.; Brady, L.-M.; Davey, C. (2011) *Guidelines for Research with Children and Young People*. London: NCB.

Shonkoff, J.P.; Phillips, D. (2000) *From Neurons to Neighbourhoods: The Science of Early Childhood Development*. New York: National Academy Press.

Siraj-Blatchford, I.; Clarke, P. (2003) *Supporting Identity, Diversity and Language in the Early Years*. Maidenhead: Open University Press.

Sixsmith, J.; Gabhainn, S.; Fleming, C.; O'Higgins, S. (2007) Children's, Parents' and Teachers' Perceptions of Child Well-being. *Health Education*, 107(6): 511–23.

Smethers, S.; Cook, G; Burstow, B. et al. (2010) 'Encouraging the bond between children and grandparents (139kb)' in *Nursing & Residential Care* 12(8): 364–365.

SMIRA (2007) *Selective Mutism Information and Research Association*. Available from http://groups.yahoo.com/group/smiratalk. Accessed 13 November 2012.

Smith, A. (2002) Interpreting and Supporting Participation Rights: Contributions from Sociocultural Theory. *International Journal of Children's Rights*, 10: 73–88.

Speech Disorder UK (2010) *Selective Mutism*. Available from www.speechdisorder.co.uk/Selective-Mutism.html. Accessed 10 April 2010.

Statham, J.; Chase, E. (2010) *Childhood Well-being: A Brief Overview*. Loughborough: Childhood Well-being Research Centre. Also available from www.education.gov.uk/publications/eOrderingDownload/Child-Wellbeing-Brief.pdf. Accessed 3 January 2013.

Strachan, R. and Tallant, C. (1995) 'The importance of framing: A pragmatic approach to risk assessment' in *Probation Journal* 42: 202–207.

Strazdins, L.; Lucas, N.; Shipley, M.; Mathews, B.; Berry, H.L.; Rodgers, B.; Davies, A. (2011) *Parent and Child Well-being and the Influence of Work and Family Arrangements: A Three Cohort Study*. FaHCSIA Social Policy Research Paper no. 44, http://papers.ssrn.com/sol3/papers.cfm?abstract_id=2185703. Accessed 13 July 2013.

Stringer, E.T. (1999) *Action Research: A Handbook for Practitioners*. Newbury Park, CA: Sage.

Sumsion, J. (2005) *Male Teachers in Early Childhood: Issues and Case Study. Early Childhood Research Quarterly*, 20(1): 109–23.

Systems of Early Education/Care and Professionalisation in Europe (Seepro) 2010 Barbara Budrich, Leverkusen.

Tabors, P. (1997) *One Child, Two Languages*. Baltimore, MD: Paul H. Brookes.

Tang, S.; Coley, R.; Votruba-Drzal, E. (2012) Low-Income Families' Selection of Childcare for Their Young Children. *Children and Youth Services Review*, 34: 2002–11.

Taratukhina, M.S.; Polyakova, M.N.; Berezina, T.A.; Notkina, N.A.; Sheraizina, R.M.; Borovkov, M.I. (2006) *Early Childhood Care and Education in the Russian Federation*. Background paper prepared for the *Education for All Global Monitoring Report 2007*. UNESCO.

Taylor, B.J. (2010) *Professional Decision Making in Social Work*. Exeter: Learning Matters.

Teater, B. (2010) *An Introduction to Applying Social Work Theories and Methods*. Maidenhead: Open University Press.

Tett, L.; Riddell, S. (2006) *Gender and Teaching: Where Have All the Men Gone?* Edinburgh: Dunedin Academic Press.

Trawick, M. (1990) *Notes on Love in a Tamil Family*. Berkeley: University of California Press.

Trodd, L.; Chivers, L. (2011) *Interprofessional Working in Practice: Learning and Working Together for Children and Families*. Maidenhead: Open University Press.

Underdown, A. (2007) *Young Children's Health and Well-being*. Maidenhead: Open University Press.

United Nations (2011) *The Millennium Development Goals Report*. Available from www.un.org/millenniumgoals/pdf/%282011_E%29%20MDG%20Report%202011_Book%20LR.pdf. Accessed 20 July 2013.

University of Washington (2013) *Centre for Child and Family Well-being*, http://depts.washington.edu/ccfwb/index.html. University of Washington, USA. Accessed 5 May 2013.

van Gelder, T. (2005) 'Teaching critical thinking: some lessons from cognitive science' in *College Teaching* 53(1): 41–48.

van Ijzendoorn, M.H.; Sagi, A. (1999) Cross-cultural Patterns of Attachment: Universal and Contextual Dimensions, in Cassidy, J.; Shaver, P.R. (eds) *Handbook of Attachment: Theory, Research and Clinical Applications*. London: Guilford Press.

Veenhoven, R. (2012) *World Database of Happiness*, www.worlddatabaseofhappiness.eur.nl/. Accessed 13 July 2013.

Viruru, R. (2001) Language as Colonization: The Case of Early Childhood Education. *Contemporary Issues in Early Childhood*, 2(1): 31–47.

Viruru, R.; Cannella, G. (2001) Postcolonial Ethnography, Young Children and Voice, in Grieshaber, S.; Cannella, G. (eds) *Embracing Identities and Early Childhood Education*. New York: Teachers College Press.

Vygotsky, L. (1978) *Mind in Society: The Development of Higher Psychological Processes*. Cambridge, MA: Harvard University Press.

Vygotsky, L. (1986) Thought and Language, in Kozulin, A. (trans and ed) *Thought and Language*. Cambridge, MA: MIT Press.

Vygotsky, L. (1987) [1934] Thinking and Speech, trans. N. Minick, in Rieber, R.; Carton, A. (eds) *The Collected Works of L.S. Vygotsky*, vol 1: *Problems of General Psychology*. New York: Plenum Press.

Vygotsky, L. (1997a) *The Collected Works of L.S. Vygotsky*. Vol 4 of *The History of the Development of Higher Mental Functions*, ed. Rieber, R. New York: Plenum.

Vygotsky, L. (1997b) Consciousness as a Problem for the Psychology of Behavior, in *The Collected Works of L.S. Vygotsky*, vol 3: *Problems of the Theory and History of Psychology*. New York: Plenum.

Waldfogel, J.; Craigie, T.-A.; Brooks-Gunn, J. (2010) Fragile Families and Child Wellbeing. *Future of Children*, 20(2): 87–112.

Wave Trust; DfE (Department for Education) (2013) *Conception to Age 2: The Age of Opportunity*. 2nd edn. Available from www.wavetrust.org/sites/default/files/key_publications/conception_to_age_2_-_the_age_of_opportunity_-_web_optimised.pdf. Accessed 20 July 2013.

Weems, L. (1999) Pestalozzi, Perversity, and the Pedagogy of Love, in Letts, W.J.; Sears, J.T. (eds) *Queering Elementary Education: Advancing the Dialogue about Sexualities and Schooling*. Lanham, MD: Rowman and Littlefield.

Wellard, S. (2012) Older People as Grandparents: How Public Policy Needs to Broaden Its View of Older People and the Role They Play within Families. *Quality in Ageing and Older Adults*, 13(4): 257–63.

Wenger, E. (1998) *Communities of Practice: Learning, Meaning and Identity*. Cambridge: Cambridge University Press.

WHO (World Health Organization) (1986) The Ottawa Charter for Health Promotion. World Health Organization Regional Publication for Europe Serial 44: 1–7

WHO (World Health Organization) (2007) *What Is Mental Health?*, www.who.int/features/qa/62/en/index.html. Accessed 20 July 2013.

WHO (World Health Organization) (2013) *Definitions: Emergencies*, www.who.int/hac/about/definitions/en/. Accessed 13 January 2013.

Wilkin, A.; Derrington, C.; Foster, B. (2009) *Improving the Outcomes for Gypsy, Roma and Traveller Pupils: A Literature Review*. Department for Children, Schools and Families Research Report no. DCSF-RR077.

Wittenberg, I. (2001) *Infant Observation*, 4(2): 23–35.

Woodhead, M. (2004) Foreword, in Kehily, M. (ed) *An Introduction to Childhood Studies*. Maidenhead: Open University Press.

Zaff, J.F. and Hair, E.C. (2003) 'Positive development of the self: Self-concept, self-esteem, and identity' www.childtrends.org/?publications=positive-development-of-the-self-self-concept-self-esteem-and-identity (accessed September 2013).

Index

Thank you for buying and reading this book.
If you found it helpful it would be great if you could

- tell your fellow students
- tell your lecturer
- post a review on Amazon
- tweet about it #criticalwellbeing

Find out about other books from Critical Publishing at
www.criticalpublishing.com

Follow us on Twitter
@CriticalPub